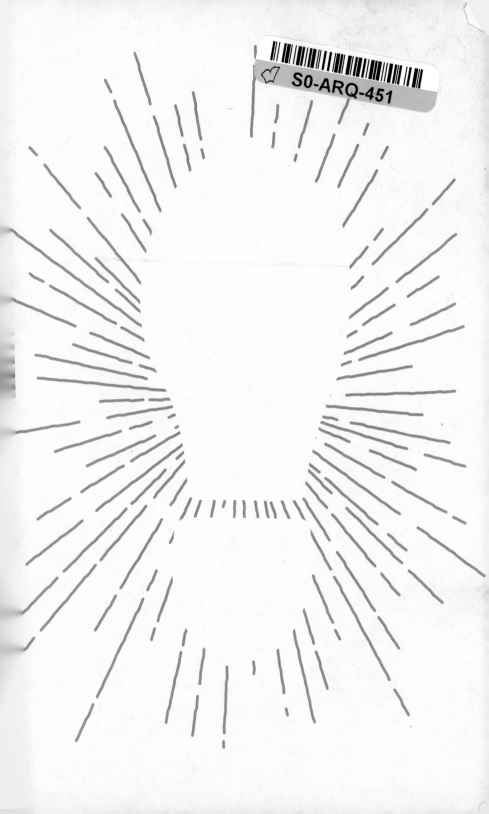

Born to WALK

the — TRANSFORMATIVE
Power OF A
PEDESTRIAN
ACT

Dan RUBINSTEIN

Published by ECW Press
665 Gerrard Street East
Toronto, Ontario, Canada M4M 1Y2
416-694-3348 / info@ecwpress.com

Editor for the press: Jennifer Knoch
Cover design: Michel Vrana

Purchase the print edition
and receive the eBook free!
For details, go to ecwpress.com/eBook.

LIBRARY AND ARCHIVES CANADA
CATALOGUING IN PUBLICATION

Rubinstein, Dan, 1973–, author
Born to walk : the transformative power
of a pedestrian act / Dan Rubinstein.

Includes bibliographical references.
ISBN 978-1-77041-419-8 (softcover)
also issued as: 978-1-77041-189-0
(hardcover), 978-1-77090-697-6 (PDF),
978-1-77090-698-3 (ePUB)

1. Walking. 2. Fitness walking. 3. Fitness
walking—Health aspects. I. Title.

RA781.65.R82 2018   613.7'176
C2017-906605-6

The publication of *Born to Walk* has been generously supported by the Canada Council
for the Arts, which last year invested $153 million to bring the arts to Canadians
throughout the country, and by the Government of Canada through the Canada
Book Fund. *Nous remercions le Conseil des arts du Canada de son soutien. L'an
dernier, le Conseil a investi 153 millions de dollars pour mettre de l'art dans la vie
des Canadiennes et des Canadiens de tout le pays. Ce livre est financé en partie par
le gouvernement du Canada.* We also acknowledge the support of the Ontario Arts
Council (OAC), an agency of the Government of Ontario, which last year funded 1,737
individual artists and 1,095 organizations in 223 communities across Ontario for a total
of $52.1 million, and the contribution of the Government of Ontario through the Ontario
Book Publishing Tax Credit and the Ontario Media Development Corporation.

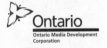

ONTARIO ARTS COUNCIL
CONSEIL DES ARTS DE L'ONTARIO
an Ontario government agency
un organisme du gouvernement de l'Ontario

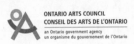

Ontario
Ontario Media Development
Corporation

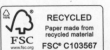

Canada Council
for the Arts

Conseil des Arts
du Canada

Canadä

PRINTED AND BOUND IN CANADA   PRINTING: MARQUIS 5 4 3 2 1

RECYCLED
Paper made from
recycled material
FSC® C103567

For Maggie, Daisy and Lisa:
My reasons to believe

FOREWORD

by Kevin Patterson

The Anthropocene era is a consequence of technology. Humans have marked the world and prevail upon it because of our tricks: the toggle-headed harpoon and the internal combustion engine and the electrical grid. These tools have allowed us to become the next asteroid. The changes they have permitted us to make upon the planet seem as unstoppable as a mass of space rock headed right for us. And they are, so long as we remain on this path, motionless and oblivious.

Motion is the subject of this book. Move, and everything changes, Dan Rubinstein writes: the way people think, how we fear, and how we understand ourselves.

A short while ago I walked along the shore of Hudson Bay. The ice had not come in yet and I watched the tundra carefully. Polar bears had come into town the week before. The reason I felt safe was that the man I was walking with carried a rifle and a GPS. People cannot outrun polar bears and we do not have the internal guidance systems of snow geese. This is the standard construction: we are the weakest animals in nature, but to compensate we have created these technologies to make ourselves formidable. And so we subdue the frontiers — because they frighten us and because we can.

It's all wrong. Humans are magnificent large mammals, as wondrous as the 200-year-old bowhead whales in Hudson Bay, or the bears, or cheetahs. What those animals are to the deep dive, to strength and the sprint, we are to the fast walk. Even if we forget it, humans are defined by our ability to walk. Our bipedalism, that is, our anatomy, not our tools, makes us uniquely efficient and fast. My grandfather claimed that over middle and long distances he could walk down a deer, so long as he could follow the track. Fresh snow in the morning meant venison by nightfall on his Peace River depression-era farm. And not a bullet need be wasted.

Hominids spent a million years on the Serengeti walking in the grass. Bruce Chatwin wrote that our bodies, from our brains to the structure of our big toes, are formed for one mission: long journeys on foot. And so long as we made them, humans understood our own capacity. But our tools have made it possible to not do the thing our bodies are optimized for. And so we forget how good we are at it, and we reach the worst possible conclusion: we are weak, unless we depend on tricks.

The Inuit on the shore of the Arctic Ocean were among the last of the great walking cultures to settle. When they came into the little towns built by the government they ceased the relentless walking that permitted them to pull a living from a land without trees or even vegetation for all but a couple months of the year. The Thule people walked from Alaska to Greenland a thousand years ago, and until Dylan went electric there were still families moving constantly between hunting sites, watching the horizon and listening to the sound of boots in the snow.

The elders who remember that life do not romanticize it. But they knew then that if they hunted as hard as they could and scoured the land and sea for food, they could keep most of their children alive. It was a dangerous life and many died of hunger and predation and cold, but they were not afraid of the land itself. There are no families living self-sufficiently on the tundra now and there probably aren't any who could. There are no people walking here or any-where on this planet who can just keep going. And because we do not walk upon the land like that anymore we cannot know it the way we did. We certainly do not feel it. Which allows us to treat it the way we do.

When we stop walking we treat the land — that is, everything — badly, and we do not spare ourselves. Twenty years ago there were no Inuit with obesity-related diabetes in the towns I worked in along the west coast of Hudson Bay. Now diabetes is exploding along with waistlines and the Inuit are quickly coming to resemble all the sed-entary people everywhere. Social nets are fraying and diabetes and suicide have become the new white bears, but with far sharper claws and larger appetites.

This is what Dan Rubinstein has written his book about: the beauty of humans walking, and what is lost when we stop. It's a gorgeous reaffirmation of our place on the planet and among our fellow creatures. He shows that, as devastating as the consequences of immobility have been, movement, and all that it brings, metabol-ically and philosophically, can be recaptured so easily. Just stand up and walk outside. Go. And keep going.

Kevin Patterson is a medical doctor who works mostly in British Columbia and Nunavut. He is the author of the novel *Consumption*, the short story collection *Country of Cold* (which won the Rogers Writers' Trust Fiction Prize), and the memoir *The Water in Between: A Journey at Sea*, and the co-editor of *Outside the Wire: The War in Afghanistan in the Words of Its Participants*.

PROLOGUE

"Perhaps walking is best imagined as an 'indicator species,' to use an ecologist's term. An indicator species signifies the health of an ecosystem, and its endangerment or diminishment can be an early warning sign of systemic trouble."

— *Rebecca Solnit,* Wanderlust: A History of Walking

"I walk in order to somatically medicate myself against the psychosis of contemporary urban living."

— *Will Self,* New York Times

The wind whipped across the frozen lake. Wet snow stung my face. It had been falling steadily since dawn, weighing down the scraggly branches of the black spruce and balsam fir that crowded the blurry shoreline. Now mid-afternoon, the flat February light was fading.

Chin tucked into jacket collar, wool toque pulled low over forehead, I shielded my eyes by studying my borrowed snowshoes, glancing up every few strides to gauge my bearings. It was a tedious way to move forward, more shackled than Shackleton. But it gave me plenty of time to think.

Lurching around the park down the street from my semi-suburban bungalow for an hour, I realized, might not have been sufficient preparation. My back ached from pulling a cheap plastic sled laden with 50 pounds of warm clothing and camping gear. I was sweaty, which can beget trouble on a winter expedition. I was thirsty: more trouble. There was chafing. And it was only the first day of a two-and-a-half-week trek. We had another 220 miles to cover.

The distance was daunting, but more so the prospect of travelling through the forest and sleeping in the snow with 60 strangers, all of whom were either Aboriginal or francophone, or both. As a unilingual Anglo urbanite accustomed to solo summer hikes and car camping, I was apprehensive about such close quarters. In fact, this whole trip charted unfamiliar turf. I knew where I was (roughly) and where we were going (vaguely), but I wasn't convinced I could get there. And, perhaps most worrisome, I had lost track of why I was trying.

There was only one certainty: it was too late to go back.

A search for direction sent me on that winter journey. The world was spinning too quickly. I needed to recalibrate. To slow down.

So I turned to an old habit.

Walking.

Until the previous year, I had followed a conventional trajectory: a happy childhood; a loving marriage; two beautiful daughters; a comfortable house; holidays on the beach; a small cushion in the bank. My career also tacked a standard path, from sports writing and newspaper reporting to a decade as a magazine editor, cresting at the top post at a respected publication. My biggest fears — environmental apocalypse, global economic collapse, runaway technology, retirement savings — were abstractions. With solid First World footing, I was confident I could muddle through, just like everyone else.

Trouble at the office catalyzed my sea change, although the restlessness was already brewing. Financial turmoil threatened to swamp the magazine industry. The non-profit where I worked responded by creating "independent and objective" content in partnership with corporate and government backers. In a business with countless shades of grey, I saw black and white. A watchdog opening the gate for wolves.

My dream job, which I had moved across the country to take, became a nightmare. Our sponsors were determined to ramp up either public support or profits, and I was aiding and abetting their newspeak. Unhinged from a sense of purpose, I felt the dissonance between what I believed in and what I was doing to pay the bills grow deafening. Energy and optimism ebbed. Simple pleasures (a home-made meal, sunset at the park) lost significance. My family soon tired of my quixotic complaints. I was trumped, rightly so, by more pressing concerns: the leaky toilet, grocery shopping, flu season.

Marooned at my desk, I swivelled round and round, drowning in digital static, a miasma of mediated boredom that, as technology critic Evgeny Morozov writes, "produces a craving for more information in order to suppress it." For months, I managed the stress by checking my email every three minutes and by taking long lunch-hour runs. Then I tore the meniscus of my right knee, painfully albeit comically, by sitting down on the ground awkwardly at a folk-music festival. The joint locked at a right angle, and after my wife helped me stand, I passed out and fell flat on the grass. It was noon. I had not been drinking (yet). On the cusp of 40, I saw this as a sign of aging. Clearly, it was time for a different approach.

A month later, trailed by an entourage of cameras, His Royal Highness Haji Al-Muhtadee Billah, the handsome crown prince of Brunei, one of the world's richest men, strode into the Carleton University Sports Medicine Clinic for a photo op as I was receiving physiotherapy. He made a beeline for my bedside and asked how I got hurt. Lying back on a mattress with interferential currents zapping my knee, surrounded by flash bulbs and zoom lenses, I did not know how to respond.

"I . . . I sat down wrong."

His Royal Highness looked at me quizzically. "In my country," he beamed, "we play a lot of badminton."

Unable to recuperate through racquet sports or running, I self-medicated with long walks whenever possible, following desire lines — paths formed by foot traffic — across railroad corridors and reedy streams. To dampen my causticity, I skipped sessions at conferences to roam around foreign cities, and assigned myself travel articles anchored by hikes. In Reno, Nevada, sweating at the spectre of another panel discussion on the ascendancy of tourism apps, I took a taxi to the trail I could see from my hotel-room window and snaked along Hunter Creek from the high desert scrublands that flank the Truckee valley to the cool Ponderosa pine meadows of Sunflower Mountain. In the rolling, frost-covered hills of Quebec's Charlevoix region, I hiked from hut to hut for four days with a group of retirees, our age and language differences irrelevant from the start. At home in Ottawa, when my daughters were in bed, I grabbed a water bottle and picked random destinations (a bridge, say, or a downtown monument), navigating by topographic feel and relishing the freedom of going with the flow. I had long been obsessed with walking, both to get from point A to point B and as a way of engaging with the world, but this was different. My habit was metastasizing. Instead of ranting about work, I ranted about walking and refused to use our beige minivan unless absolutely necessary.

Infatuated by transects people seldom experience slowly, I walked from my childhood bedroom in Toronto to my parents' off-the-grid cottage, spending four days on a commute that takes three hours in a car. It was an attempt to honour the cabin's ragged spirit, to better understand the well-worn yet never static relationship between city and countryside, between my family and me. On night two, blistered and hobbling, I was saved by the proprietor of a B&B in a reborn brick church. She drew a hot bath and handed me a cold beer. "The world is a book," she had written in jaunty white letters on a chalkboard in the kitchen, quoting St. Augustine, "and those who do not travel read only a page."

Regardless of the destination, at some point during each walk, *everything* would seem better. (Though not when I pulled up lame at a boat launch 20 kilometres shy of the cottage and borrowed a cellphone to call for a ride, giving my father the wrong coordinates, an error he never tires of mentioning.) The harmonic feeling would descend while I was in motion, and sometimes lingered — "a state in which the mind, the body, and the world are aligned," as Rebecca Solnit writes in *Wanderlust*, "as though they were three characters finally in conversation together, three notes suddenly making a chord." A chord that was still ringing in the recesses of my brain when, back at my computer, easily distracted from the tasks on my to-do lists, I began tripping over reams of fresh research into the physiological and psychological virtues of walking. The social, economic and creative possibilities too. Was this a frequency illusion, triggered by my obsession? Or a prescription for change?

Whether for transportation or recreation, walking bestows the gift of time. Done by choice, untethered from the market and wireless contraptions, it can be an act of defiance. At its most pure, walking connects us to the people and places where we are *right now*. Also, to ourselves. In the early decades of the 21st century, an era of climactic convulsions, rapacious profiteering, crushing debt, deadly "lifestyle" diseases and the attenuation of non-virtual community, these are precious commodities. They might pay tremendous dividends.

The French have a term for those who view the world through the lens of their vocation, at the expense of a broader perspective: *déformation professionnelle*. After more than 20 years as a journalist, I saw everything, foremost, as a story. Could I apply this condition to walking?

"So, what would you say," I asked Lisa, my wife, as we did the dishes one evening, "if I made walking my job? For a while?"

She bit her lip. Rinsed a wineglass. Lisa had recently traded freelance writing for stable employment, anticipating my flight of fancy.

"You'd be a warker," she said. "Or a wolker."

I took that as a yes.

Seeking specialists who also suspected that something so humble could have a profound impact on our lives, or at least enablers who were willing to listen, I contacted the people whose work I had been reading about. The epidemiologist in Glasgow investigating the links between walking and depression. The criminologist in Philadelphia assessing the impact of police officers on foot patrol. The physiological anthropologist in Japan analyzing how a walk in the woods alters our bodies at a molecular level. The ex–transportation engineer in New York City walking every street of every borough. The scientists in Toronto using a one-of-a-kind laboratory to help people remain mobile. The Brit who walked across the Middle East and Central Asia, then went home and campaigned for a seat in Parliament by tramping around his rural constituency. Admittedly, I was scratching a mid-life itch, escaping as much as approaching. But these women and men, and a couple dozen others, were rigorous and esteemed. And they agreed to share their discoveries.

This book is about the transformative properties of walking. About fissures that anyone can explore. It is the outcome of an experiment both personal and journalistic, an attempt to understand my addiction, to see how much repair might be within range.

I have tried to structure it in a logical way, exploring one main benefit of walking in each chapter. This is a problematic construction: the anecdotes, statistics and conclusions overlap and magnify one another. There are also geographic boundaries to stumble over. While I touch down in Asia, Africa and Latin America, the focus is on the United States, the United Kingdom and Canada. The cultural and economic forces that have shaped the Anglosphere (our cities and habits, our health and happiness) have incubated a distinct set of challenges.

Maturity, we are told, means accepting that the world is broken. Yet, what if some simple patches were possible? All of the people I spoke to or spent time with, outstanding in diverse fields, have demonstrated, in one way or another, that a renewed emphasis on walking, even in communities facing stacked odds, could be a small step toward somewhere better. That my fix just might be a fix.

Generations of writers have gone down this road. Wordsworth, Thoreau, Solnit, Chatwin and scores of others have crafted lyrical poems, essays and books about the power of walking. I bow at their feet. These classics are more relevant now than ever, and they have kindled a resurgence. In 2014 alone, French philosopher Frédéric Gros published a manifesto about the subversive ability of walking to mine the "mystery of presence"; British author Nick Hunt retraced the 80-year-old footsteps of scholar Patrick Leigh Fermor across Europe on a quest to find what remains of the kindness of strangers; historian Matthew Algeo looked back at an era when competitive walking was America's most popular spectator sport; and naturalist Trevor Herriot embarked on a prairie pilgrimage, wielding "a metaphysics of hope against the dogma that we are aimless wanderers in a world whose chaotic surface is the sum total of reality." This indispensable paper trail gave my ideas shape and scope.

One of the first guides I talked to was a doctor named Stanley Vollant, the first Aboriginal surgeon from Quebec. A son of the Innu nation, Vollant was striving to inspire hope among Canada's indigenous peoples by leading group hikes hundreds of miles long, reviving the routes and rhythms of his ancestors. There was a walk coming up. He invited me to tag along.

At the time, I was bogged down by work and domestic responsibilities. But our conversation continued to resonate. "When you begin a journey, you don't know why," Vollant had said sagely. "The trail will show you the way."

My employer held its annual gala a month before Christmas. The country's corporate and political elite congregated in the grand hall of a museum amid towering totem poles and an arcing wall of floor-to-ceiling windows that frame a view of the federal government's Gothic revival fortress on the far side of the river. Making small talk with big people is a smart way to climb ladders. But I missed the party. Earlier that day, an orthopedic surgeon had performed an arthroscopy on my injured knee, trimming a torn flap of cartilaginous tissue from the crescent-shaped pad that gives the joint structural integrity.

After three weeks of rest and rehab, I quit my job and assembled a pulk for hauling gear. Then I went walking.

one

BODY

"Each step we take is an arrested plunge, a collapse averted, a disaster braked. . . . We perform it daily: a two-beat miracle — an iambic teetering, a holding on and letting go."

— *Paul Salopek*, National Geographic

"Do not judge your neighbour until you walk two moons in his moccasins."

— *Cheyenne proverb*

Dr. Stanley Vollant was desperate for sleep. He flew to Rotorua, New Zealand, for an indigenous health conference in October 2007, landing drained and depressed after a full day of travel. His second wife had just left him, taking their toddler son. Despite stellar credentials, including a term as president of the Quebec Medical Association, he was overwhelmed by shifts in the operating room, clinics in remote communities and his duties as director of the University of Ottawa's Aboriginal medicine program. Vollant, a charismatic role model with modest roots, had recently put a gun in his mouth and come close to pulling the trigger.

At his hotel in Rotorua, a friend recommended going for a short run to ease the jet lag.

"I'm so tired," Vollant protested.

"You're a marathon runner, Stan. Go for maybe 15, 20 minutes."

"I don't have any strength. I don't feel good."

"Go."

Too weak to argue, Vollant laced up his shoes and jogged into the volcanic valley on the outskirts of town. The primordial landscape, a paradise of geysers and hot springs and bubbling mud pools, was energizing. He had the sensation that he was flying.

During the run, which stretched into three effortless hours, Vollant had a vivid daydream. He was walking in a faraway place. He did not know where.

One night after returning home, back in his rut, he turned on the television. A man was talking about El Camino de Santiago, the popular Christian pilgrimage in Spain. Vollant, who believes in the values but not the hierarchies of Catholicism, looked at his bedside table. On top sat a book, bought five years earlier and pushed aside unread: *The Pilgrimage*, by Paulo Coelho, a novel inspired by the author's experiences on the Camino. The Aboriginal part of Vollant's brain pulled rank on his Cartesian training. He knew what to do next.

The following spring, still squeezed for time, Vollant set out to complete the Camino at an ambitious pace — 26 miles a day for 18 days. Most people take nearly twice as long. "I'm a marathon runner," he told his girlfriend before departing. "I can do this."

She lifted his 45-pound red backpack. An avid long-distance hiker, she never carried more than 20 pounds. "Stan," she warned, "you're going to feel every ounce of this."

"Honey, I'm a strong man. For me, 45 pounds is nothing."

After his first day in the Spanish Pyrenees, Vollant had a half-dozen blisters. With each step, he felt every *fucking* ounce of his pack.

Stubbornly, he continued without shedding any gear, even though there was too much snow to use his tent, forcing him to bunk in communal *albergues*. After 12 days, shivering uncontrollably, he stumbled toward a small-town hotel, fainting twice before reaching the front desk. A long bath and a restaurant meal restored some strength. He pared down his pack in the morning and, ignoring the festering blisters, walked for another two days. Excruciating pain in his toes and an expanding red spot on his shin finally convinced him to take a train to León, where he went straight to the hospital. Doctors diagnosed the infection — fasciitis, a precursor to flesh-eating disease — and pumped intravenous antibiotics into his blood for five days. "Go back to Canada," he was instructed at discharge. Instead, because doctors do make the worst patients, he returned to the Camino. Which is where the second vision came.

In a barnlike refuge, with the mountain wind blowing bursts of rain in through gaps around the doors, Vollant had a dream as clear as HDTV, right down to his red backpack. This time, he was walking in a familiar forest with Aboriginal youth and elders. They were abstaining from alcohol and drugs, eating healthy food, talking about their cultures, healing bodies, minds and spirits.

When he awoke, covered in sweat, Vollant described what he had seen to a fellow pilgrim. "What am I supposed to do?" he asked. "Why? How?"

"Your people believe that dreams have meaning," André, a Frenchman, reminded him. "They are the call of destiny."

Vollant came home from Spain wondering whether he was crazy. Walking across a chunk of Canada was an intriguing idea. Maybe when he retired. When he had more time and money. When his children, a pair of daughters from his first marriage, and his young son, Xavier, didn't need him around so much. The journey in his dream would require the better part of a year. He could take time off work to attend medical conferences. But not for this.

Nonetheless, friends and relatives encouraged Vollant. Like him, they saw an escalating need for the type of project he had in mind. Not in the future. Now. Thus divined, bolstered by a compelling creation myth, the Innu Meshkenu — Innu Road — took shape. A six-year, 3,800-mile series of walks, in all seasons, between every Aboriginal community in Quebec and Labrador, and a few in

Ontario and New Brunswick. Vollant wanted to demonstrate the power of believing in yourself. That any change was possible, as long as you approached it with perseverance. And that walking, at its core a physical tonic, was an ideal way to start.

Canada's 1.4 million Aboriginal people are a diverse group. Urban and rural, rich and poor, digitally savvy and subsistence hunters, doctors and dropouts, in harmony with the earth and struggling into the gale, there are vast differences within and between southern First Nations, northern Inuit, mixed-race Métis and the 16,000 or so eastern Innu. Demographically, however, when you compare them to the country's non-Aboriginal population, the statistics reveal an alarming truth: many endure health challenges on par with people in the developing world, despite living in one of the wealthiest nations on the planet.

Aboriginal men and women die an average of seven years earlier than other Canadians. The infant mortality rate is 1.5 times higher. (Among Inuit, life expectancy is 15 years lower than the national average and the infant mortality rate is four times higher.) Aboriginal people are 1.5 times more likely to have at least one chronic medical condition, such as diabetes, high blood pressure or arthritis. Fifty-six percent of First Nations children between the ages of two and 17 on reserves are overweight or obese, compared to 26 percent of non-Aboriginal children, the Public Health Agency of Canada reported in 2009. A year later, in a report called "A Perfect Storm," Canada's Heart and Stroke Foundation issued a warning about heart disease, citing skyrocketing national rates of high blood pressure (a 77 percent jump), diabetes (45 percent) and obesity (18 percent) between 1994 and 2005. Unless something changes, cardiovascular emergencies will overload the country's health-care system. Aboriginal people, the foundation declared, are already experiencing "a full-blown crisis."

Statistics on alcoholism, substance abuse, incarceration (4 percent of the population, 25 percent of inmates) and suicide — the most common cause of death for Aboriginals aged 44 and under — show the severity of this crisis. And there are signs that it will deepen.

Canada's Aboriginal population is the youngest and fastest-growing demographic group in the country, increasing by 20 percent between 2006 and 2011, versus 5.2 percent among non-Aboriginals. The median age is 28, compared to 41 in the rest of the country, and almost half of all Aboriginals are 24 or younger. These numbers have dire implications. If today's health inequalities are not addressed, the social and financial costs will balloon out of control.

Centuries of economic and educational apartheid, and the lost generations abused by Church and State at residential schools — the persistent echoes of colonization — have led us here. Acute concerns abound: decrepit housing, domestic violence, toxic water. Triage is required in many of the communities that Innu Meshkenu passes through. And while the project emphasizes the importance of mental and spiritual strength, and the need to re-establish a connection to the land, to tradition and to one another, as any physician will tell you, it's tough to go far without a healthy body.

Vollant's first walk, in October 2010, was a 385-mile solo hike west along the St. Lawrence River, from the Innu reserve in Natashquan, Quebec, to Baie-Comeau, the city closest to Pessamit, the village where he is from, about 370 miles northeast of Montreal. Flying to the starting point in a small plane, he stared down at the terrain he would soon be travelling, questioning once more his sanity. On a map, 18 miles per day seemed reasonable. From 15,000 feet, it looked deadly. Maybe if he went to the nursing station in Natashquan he would be put in a straitjacket and locked away? But then he landed and saw cardboard signs written in Montagnais, his language, welcoming him home. Route 138, the paved highway that extends east from Montreal, terminates just past Natashquan. White people call this the end of the road. To Innu, it is the beginning.

Vollant's momentum has snowballed since he walked to Baie-Comeau in 23 days, with supporters literally coming out of the woods to set up tents and cook meals of moose and salmon. He completed seven more walks in 2011 and 2012, most lasting two to three weeks, distances ranging from 200 to 450 miles. A couple were short excursions, such as the two-day march from Wôlinak to Odanak in southern Quebec in September 2012 for the opening of an Aboriginal college, a trek that drew 150 participants. Even the long walks have been getting more crowded. In some ways, they're similar to *Survivor*, I would discover, only the goal is to get more people *onto* the island.

The winter 2013 leg began in Manawan, an Atikamekw reserve at the end of an icy 55-mile-long gravel road, a four-hour drive north of Montreal. Three months after my knee surgery, I got a ride there with a pair of Québécois walkers, and after I insisted we take a shortcut where the snowbanks soon reached the roof of our hatchback, we retreated to the plowed route and arrived a little late, although not too late for the feast in the elementary school gymnasium. The festivities would begin on "Indian time."

This can be a derogatory term, used to connote an aversion to schedules. But re-appropriated by Aboriginals, ingrained within a long history of adhering to the seasons or the weather or the migratory patterns of animals, not the confines of calendar and clock, it is really, in the words of Ojibwe author Drew Hayden Taylor, "an enigmatic idea based on a uniquely cultural relationship with time. Simply put, things happen when they happen. . . . The universe has its own heartbeat, and who are we to speed it up or slow it down?" As I watched a slideshow of photos from previous Innu Meshkenu walks while listening to seven men pound a drum and chant, European time already felt out of whack.

Vollant was still in transit on the eve of the expedition, en route from the Université de Montréal, where he lectures at the medical school when not working as a locum — or stand-in — surgeon throughout the province. The logistics were in the calm, calloused hands of his project manager, Jean-Charles Fortin, an outdoor recreation and adventure tourism instructor at Université du Québec à Chicoutimi. "I grew up in the Mohawk community of Kanesatake, Quebec," he told the group when we gathered on folding chairs in the gym for the first of many circles, confiding to me later that this introduction is mostly a "social lubricant" — he *might* have some Métis blood. Fortin, with his shoulder-length dark hair and shiny dark eyes, does have a problem-solving, those-are-not-my-rules attitude. A diehard mountain biker, he knows all the backwoods trails around Kanesatake. During the month-long armed standoff between the Canadian army and Mohawk warriors over the expansion of a golf course on tribal land in 1990, before the proliferation of cellphones and digital cameras, he ferried rolls of film and notepads around police barricades for reporters, charging $100 per trip. At the end of the conflict, he had enough cash for a new car.

Fortin found spare rooms in a local's basement for my Québécois companions and me — beds and breakfast from a family without much to spare — and we reconvened outside the school in the morning. My pulk was packed and secured to a padded waist belt with nylon rope fed through cross-hatched aluminum poles. About 300 people came out for the ceremonial departure. There was only one problem: no Vollant. He was making a presentation to students in the gym, a cornerstone of every Innu Meshkenu stop. We stood around and waited, stamping our feet to stay warm. This turned out to be a blessing, because there was in fact a second problem. Fat snowflakes were accumulating and melting on my stuff sacks; my bedding and clothing were getting soaked. Everyone else had a plastic tarp, cinched tight with bungee cords, to keep their gear dry. Despite weeks of planning and provisioning, despite the shelf of tarps in my garage, despite Lisa's suggestion that a waterproof cover might come in handy, I did not bring one.

My aluminum poles clanged like the bell at a railroad crossing as I ran down the hill to Manawan's gas station / general store, the only retailer in town. Rushing up and down the aisles, which were thick with shoppers on a weekday morning, I saw no tarps. Trying not to panic, I broke out my broken French.

"*Je cherche pour un* . . . tarp," I said to a young employee, extending my arms wide to compensate for my woeful pronunciation and Grade 9 vocabulary. "*Un grand* tarp *plastique. Pour un bateau?*"

He shook his head. Maybe because boating season was months away. Maybe because the short, sweaty guy in front of him clearly required the type of assistance that a general store cannot provide.

Outside, a man wearing a hunting cap was admiring the sleek lines of my baby-blue $20 sled (purchased at a Canadian Tire outlet with a bountiful selection of tarps). *"Le marcher avec le docteur,"* I mumbled, then repeated my *"plastique, bateau"* appeal. Amazingly, he nodded. After a series of hand gestures, I understood that Mario would meet me at the school with a tarp. Or that I was a fool, and he sincerely wished I would not freeze to death in the bush. Not long after I got back to the staging area, Mario appeared with a grey-green tarp large enough to gift-wrap a rowboat. I gave him a $20 bill, shook his large hand with both of mine and managed to cover my gear by the time Vollant arrived.

Sweet grass and sage were burned, elders recited prayers in Atikamekw (an Algonquian language) and French, and then the doctor addressed the crowd. Six feet tall and a little over his running weight at 195 pounds, Vollant had light brown skin, a broad Roman nose and kind eyes. With his long, greying hair tucked away in a bun, the 48-year-old looked like a cross between Kobe Bryant and Mario Lemieux. "My ancestors walked on this land for thousands of years. I am doing as they did," he said in English with a warm, rich French accent, like narrator Roch Carrier in the National Film Board's classic animated film *The Sweater*. "These walks are all about individual and community empowerment. People start to believe in their own dreams and become more of a presence in their own lives." Old and young, women and men nodded, several with tears in their eyes. In an airport hotel banquet room, these words might sound cheap. On the rez, they had heft.

Well-wishers lined both sides of the path and showered us with handclasps and high-fives as we walked single-file into the woods. I stuck close to Vollant. He told me about his feverish vision on the Camino. Then the trail narrowed and I fell behind.

Innu Meshkenu participants are supposed to be autonomous.

The route is discussed in advance, and signs are planted in the snow to indicate how far you have travelled and where to turn. You carry enough water and food for the day, and Fortin's logisticians rumble back and forth on snowmobiles to make sure nobody is in danger. "Our job," one told me, "is to keep you alive." We were starting soft: an 11-mile kickoff, with backcountry cabins for cooking and eating the first two nights. I was warm, my knee was fine. Still, the pulk and snowshoes were cumbersome, and by afternoon I was weakening.

The wind intensified as I walked atop a meandering river and onto the icy expanse of Lac Mazana. Clumps of snow froze in my beard. Alone in a squall, embarking on my first winter camping trip, away from my daughters for the longest span of their short lives, I wondered whether my search was a fantasy. What on earth would I find?

And then I spotted smoke wafting skyward. Even better: bear hugs from brawny guys I had met only that morning. Welcome to camp one.

With help from the 15-person support crew, men were setting up small galvanized-steel wood stoves inside canvas tents and fitting together sections of chimney pipe. Women spread fir and cedar boughs over the snow for bedding. Evergreen needles and burning hardwood scented the air. The tea and soup were ready, Fortin told me, though I was advised not to take too much. Turkey fajitas were on the menu for supper.

A wiry grey-haired man from Manawan beckoned me into one of the cabins. I hung my wet layers by the fire, donned down pants and a puffy blue parka that Lisa calls "Fleischman" (the anxiety-riddled Jewish doctor from Manhattan who moves to an Alaskan outpost in the TV show *Northern Exposure*), and followed Jean-Alfred Flamand back out. The 53-year-old moved and spoke slowly at the send-off feast. He seemed tired, frail. Here, after setting a fast pace across the lake, the guy everybody called Napech — "youngest of the elders" in Atikamekw — was downing dead trees with a chainsaw and splitting rounds of wood with one hand.

The 45 walkers ranged in age from 13 to 67, and two-thirds were women. Most were from the Atikamekw nation. For centuries, their ancestors were semi-nomadic hunter-gatherers in Quebec's upper Saint-Maurice River basin. Manawan did not get year-round road access until 1973. Another main village, Wemotaci, only became a permanent settlement in the 1970s. Atikamekw culture remains strong: children learn their mother tongue before French, and hunting is a common activity. But growing up on the reserve presents challenges, including an above-average risk of obesity and diabetes, and myriad ailments associated with a sedentary lifestyle, poor diet and poverty.

Vollant used to drive his SUV or fly into isolated communities to talk to children about the virtues of physical activity, and dreams, but his message wasn't getting through. His way of life appeared out of reach. Now he approaches on foot, taking days or weeks to get there, and kids are more likely to listen. "We want walking to become, again, a social norm in native communities," Fortin had said to me in Manawan. "We want people who take their ATVs 300 metres to go to the grocery store to look stupid. Right now, it's the opposite."

Today, in much of the world, especially North America, we don't walk nearly as much as we used to. Lisa and I may be part of the first generation in 1,000 years to raise children with shorter life expectancies than their parents. Obesity and inactivity are the main culprits. In the U.S., where sidewalks are often the domain of immigrants, the elderly and the poor, people walk less than in any other industrialized nation. "Americans are in the habit of never walking," the Duke of Orléans and future king of France, Louis Philippe, said in 1798, "if they can ride." More recently, a pedometer study showed that Australian adults average about 9,700 steps each day, Swiss 9,650, Japanese 7,150, Canadians 6,700 and Americans 5,100. In Manchester, Kentucky, a town in the Appalachian foothills where 52 percent of adults are obese, double the national average, the *Washington Post* photographed a 12-year-old girl getting a ride to the school bus stop at the end of her driveway.

"The decline of walking," Tom Vanderbilt writes in *Traffic: Why We Drive the Way We Do (and What It Says About Us)*, "has become a full-blown public health nightmare." In this regard at least, 125 years after the massacre at Wounded Knee, Americans and Canadians are on common ground with the people whose land we stole.

After day one's slog, historical wrongs and pedometer counts are the last thing on my mind. All I want is a place to stow my pack. "Take a space in the reporters' tent," says Fortin, nodding toward an open flap. Inside, sitting beside the stove, Mathieu-Robert Sauvé, a fit, bespectacled 50-something writer and videographer from Montreal, is rubbing Vaseline on his feet, a veteran manoeuvre. He completed the previous winter's walk and has been writing about Vollant in French for five years already. Smiling wearily, he shoves his duffel bag into the corner to make room.

"Who else is in here?" I ask, relieved to be bunking with somebody fluently bilingual, even if he is my rival (and has home snow advantage).

"Stanley will be there," says Sauvé, pointing to a pile of gear, including the red backpack, now stuffed with medical supplies. "And his cousin" — police officer Éric Hervieux — "against the far wall." I move Vollant's backpack and unfurl my Therm-a-Rest. Journalists are told not to sleep with their subjects, but nobody has ever cautioned me about sleeping *beside* someone.

Hervieux — stocky, stoic and unintentionally intimidating — ducks into the tent, greets me with a silent nod and lies down for a nap. He lives and works in Pessamit and arrived in Manawan with Vollant in the middle of the night. Our chief is not in camp right now. Vollant took a *motoneige* back to town to prepare for a phone call with the Canada Revenue Agency. Since starting Innu Meshkenu, he has been trading shifts as a surgeon for time on the trail, and his salary has plummeted. This has made it difficult to pay his bills. He is so far behind on support payments to his ex-wives, both doctors, that his passport was taken away — the kind of concern that tends to fade in the forest.

Broiling inside Fleischman, I leave the tent to seek out a chore. It doesn't matter what kind of shape you're in or how tired you are — even if it's frying bannock or mending moccasins, Fortin's orientation talk had made it clear that when you get to camp, you work.

After taking a few ineffectual swipes at a log with a large axe, I settle into my five-foot-four city-slicker niche: carrying branches to the women and distributing kindling to the men. The more I move, the more energy I feel. Around me, everyone is busy. All of this bustle demonstrates a counterintuitive truth: one of the best treatments for fatigue is moderate activity. Especially if it doesn't feel like exercise.

In 1950, London physiologist Richard Doll published a paper in the *British Medical Journal* illuminating the link between cigarettes and lung cancer. A pioneer in the use of medical statistics, Doll had suspected that road tar or occupational factors might be behind the rising incidence of the disease in the U.K. since the 1930s. But after he and several colleagues completed research projects, they found the smoking gun. It wasn't until 1954 that British health minister Iain Macleod endorsed the findings at a press conference — while chain-smoking at the podium. Kowtowing to the tobacco lobby, only decades later did governments around the world begin their campaigns to curb cigarette use. Big Tobacco buried the truth. Billions of dollars were at risk.

Doll played a behind-the-scenes role in this drama. One of his contemporaries, London doctor Jerry Morris, has an equally hidden historical profile. Which is a shame, because at the same time that we were slowly awakening to the dangers of cigarettes, we had no idea how closely physical activity and health were connected. And judging by the glut of proprietary dieting programs, body-altering surgeries and other commercial cures, we are still in denial.

After serving as a military doctor in India during World War II, Liverpool-born, Glasgow-raised Morris returned to London. Alongside lung cancer, incidence of heart attacks had been increasing, and nobody could figure out why. Morris had a hunch that occupation could be a factor. He led a large study looking at heart-attack rates among Londoners in a variety of professions: transportation workers, teachers, letter carriers and others. The transportation data was ready first, in 1949, and revealed a marked difference between bus drivers and conductors, men from the same social class. Drivers, who sat all day, had more heart attacks; conductors climbed up and down the stairs on double-decker buses. Morris waited nervously for the rest of the data. When it landed, he compared mailmen to clerks. The results confirmed his hypothesis. "Coronary Heart-Disease and Physical Activity of Work," published in the *Lancet* in 1953, was the first major scientific paper to assert that "regular physical exercise could be one of the 'ways of life' that promote health." Morris has been called "the man who invented exercise."

In a society where physical toil was rapidly being stripped from the daily routines of white-collar city dwellers, it took a number-crunching doctor to assert a truth that now seems preposterously self-evident. Swayed by Doll's work and his own studies, Morris quit smoking and started jogging. "Exercise normalizes the workings of the body," he told a reporter in 2009, still regularly doing research out of his office at the London School of Hygiene & Tropical Medicine. "Humans were meant to keep active." He died two months later at the age of 99.

To commemorate Morris, please stand. Push off with one of your feet and swing that leg forward. When your heel strikes the ground, roll your foot until the toes make contact. Now do the same thing with the other leg. And repeat. A few more times. Sounds simple, if you're able-bodied. It isn't.

Upright ambulation began long before our ancestors evolved into *Homo sapiens* some 200,000 years ago. Anthropologists are not sure exactly when and why the early hominins that predated *Homo erectus* and Neanderthals developed bipedalism. Fossils and skulls found over the past few decades have indicated that we started walking on two feet around 6 million years ago and became mostly bipedal around 4 million years ago. When East Africa's grasslands began to spread, roughly 2 million years ago, we became fully bipedal — the only species of primate to make this leap.

Our bodies adapted to help us navigate the savannah. The prehensile feet that clung to trees in prehistoric forests were last season's model. We had to cover large, open spaces to find food and escape predators. Standing upright also helped us reach fruits on low branches. In *The Descent of Man*, Charles Darwin wrote that we needed to free up our hands and arms, which "could hardly have become perfect enough to have manufactured weapons, or to have hurled stones and spears with a true aim, as long as they were habitually used for locomotion." Kent State University anthropologist C. Owen Lovejoy expanded on Darwin's ideas and linked bipedalism to monogamy. Males needed their hands to carry food back to females who were taking care of babies; they became sole providers. Other theories, that we began walking upright to see over tall grasses, or to minimize exposure to the sun, or to facilitate male phallic display, have been largely discredited.

To move efficiently, our ape ancestors developed an inverted pendulum stride, a feat of balance and coordination. "Using a stiff leg as a point of support, the body swings up and over it in an arc," Jennifer Ackerman explains in *National Geographic*, "so that the potential energy gained in the rise roughly equals the kinetic energy generated in the descent. By this trick the body stores and recovers so much of the energy used with each stride that it reduces its own workload by as much as 65 percent." We lacked speed and strength, but this gait gave us stamina, and an edge over other species.

Around 60,000 years ago, our forebears trickled north out of Africa. After loitering around the Middle East for a while, some hung a left toward Europe (my kin), while others fanned out across Asia (Vollant's people). To help us process all the new information we were encountering as we spread around the globe, our brains grew. The great migration reached the Bering Land Bridge about 20,000 years ago, and the Americas experienced their first real estate boom. But nobody stayed put for long. Seasonal foraging and overland trading did not cease, and famines, war and persecution continue to trigger massive waves of exodus. We may have harnessed the power of horses, trains and cars, but walking is survival. When the going gets tough, we get going.

Neuroscientists have a pretty good picture of what happens inside our heads to make us walk. The Brain from Top to Bottom, a website produced by Montreal's McGill University, offers a thorough description. Voluntary movement starts in the motor cortex, at the rear of the brain's frontal lobe. The motor cortex communicates with other parts of the brain, including the visual cortex and cerebellum, and the vestibular system, the balancing apparatus in our inner ear — a feedback loop of electrochemical information about the body's position in space, the goal to be attained, an appropriate strategy for attaining it and memories of past strategies. The cerebellum, tucked beneath the back of the brain, is like an air-traffic controller, regulating the details of each motion. Neurons in the motor cortex have long extensions, or axons, that descend into the spinal cord. As we evolved from quadrupeds into an upright species, our bodies realigned into a column, with the long, forward-tilting primate pelvis taking on the squat, vertical form it has today. The skull also changed; the foramen magnum, the hole through which the motor cortex axons connect to the spinal cord, shifted from the back of the skull to the bottom. These axons transit information to motor neurons in the spinal cord via connecting synapses, and the motor neurons send impulses to our muscles, causing them to contract. In total, about 100 million neurons fire, and your foot — an intricate structure with 26 bones, 33 articulations, 111 ligaments and more than 20 muscles — begins to lift.

Coordinated movements are largely the result of patterns, which are easier for the brain to retain and retrieve than individual actions. After babies learn to walk — a progression that requires sufficient strength, balance, practice and brain development — the behaviour eventually becomes automatic because we follow the same process millions of times. (Narrow birth canals were another by-product of evolution, giving us unique brains that grow dramatically outside the womb, to minimize the risk of getting stuck during labour. As a result, we need more care than other primates as newborns, and our immature brains need more time to master the complexities of self-directed movement.)

Once we're mobile and toddle across the living room a few hundred times, the motor cortex can tune out. "A lot of basic movements never make it to your brain," says Harvard biologist and locomotion expert Daniel Lieberman. "A runner doesn't have to tell her legs what to do each time she takes a step, because there are basic reflexes that tell the legs what to do." When the brain does kick in, it needs only 5 to 10 milliseconds to sense a stimulus, such as a slip on a patch of ice, and another 30 or so milliseconds to make our muscles react.

This automation, argue Australian father-son researchers Rick and Mac Shine, an evolutionary biologist and a neuroscientist respectively, frees up the brain to concentrate on more complex matters. Walking upright, they theorize in a 2014 paper, made our species smarter. When we started to stand on two legs, "our brains were overwhelmed with the complicated challenge of keeping our balance," says Mac, "and the best kind of brain to have was one that didn't waste its most powerful functions on controlling routine tasks. . . . So, humans are smart because we have automated the routine tasks, and thus, can devote our most potent mental faculties to deal with new, unpredictable challenges."

The human brain may be our most sophisticated feature, but it is only a small part of the planet's most complex machine. Thousands more internal mechanisms keep us walking. My favourite, with a nod to my sitting injury, is synovial fluid. When you move, the yolk-like liquid in your knees and other common joints (hips, ankles, shoulders) gets warmer and thinner, and more easily absorbed by cartilage. This "human motor oil" does more than act as a lubricant. It supplies oxygen and nutrients to the cells that maintain a healthy cartilaginous matrix. Once infused with the liquid, cartilage swells like a sponge, cushioning against compression. When squeezed, fluid and metabolic wastes are discharged. Without this cycle, the cartilage deteriorates, and the joint doesn't operate as smoothly as it should.

Your heart also needs exercise to remain healthy. Through regular exertion, it grows larger, stronger and more efficient, pumping out a greater volume of blood with each beat. This blood carries vital oxygen to your muscles. Your body fuels this activity by consuming stored carbohydrates and fat, preventing plaque buildup in your arteries and burning calories that would otherwise add weight. Clear arteries and a lean physique allow the heart to pump at a lower pressure, which reduces the strain on the organ. All this work raises your temperature slightly, which releases hormones such as epinephrine and glucagon, helping muscles absorb energy. Endorphins flow into your brain, blocking pain signals and producing feelings of pleasure. Levels of insulin, which makes the body absorb glucose from blood, drop. Most people, if they remain hydrated and eat right, can walk for hours with virtually no wear and tear.

Evolutionary compromises have left us in the lurch in some respects. The vertebral column, originally an arch, developed a pair of S curves, in the lower and upper back. These help us maintain balance while walking but aren't so great at bearing weight. Delicate vertebral disks can slip or squish together. More than 15 million Americans go to the doctor with back pain every year. Bipedalism also imposes forces equal to several multiples of our body weight on the knee and foot, says physical anthropologist Bruce Latimer, resulting in injuries. Meniscus tears and arthritic knees are commonplace. A flat foot can lead to fatigue fractures; too much of an arch can inflame ligaments or cause plantar fasciitis. "We have a desire to see the story of bipedalism as a linear, progressive thing, one model improving on another, all evolving toward perfection in *Homo sapiens*," says paleontologist Will Harcourt-Smith. "But evolution doesn't evolve toward anything. It's a messy affair, full of diversity and dead ends."

Bad backs and blown knees notwithstanding, the therapeutic properties of travelling around on your feet are powerful. By using our bioelectrical, biochemical, respiratory, muscular, cardiovascular and skeletal systems in such a controlled manner, our body gets the workout it needs to function optimally. This measured exertion protects people from obesity, coronary disease, heart attacks, strokes and Type 2 diabetes, which is a leading cause of vision loss, kidney failure and limb amputation. Walking builds bone mass, strengthens the muscles in your arms and legs, and gives your joints better range of motion. It enhances your balance, preventing falls, and eases back pain (most of the time, anyway). It lowers the risk of glaucoma by reducing intraocular pressure. Tests on mice have shown that brisk walking may slow the death of light-sensitive retinal cells by stimulating production of a protein called BDNF, a discovery that could help prevent macular degeneration, the leading cause of blindness among the elderly.

The take-away: walking keeps you healthy and helps you live longer. Or, as Hippocrates said, "walking is man's best medicine."

The internet is flooded with academic papers that support this ancient aphorism. Rather than deconstruct the corporeal rewards of walking from head to toe, let's focus on a pair of survey studies. In 2008, two scientists from University College London did a meta-analysis of walking research published between 1970 and 2007 in English-language, peer-reviewed journals. They looked at almost 4,300 articles and concentrated on 18. These studies, which investigated the well-being and walking habits of about 460,000 people, lasted an average of 11.3 years. A comprehensive range of health characteristics and events were considered: age, smoking, alcohol use, heart attack, heart failure, coronary artery bypass surgery, stroke and death. The analysis, as summarized by Harvard Medical School, determined that walking "reduced the risk of cardiovascular events by 31 percent, and it cut the risk of dying during the study period by 32 percent. These benefits were equally robust in men and women. Protection was evident even at distances of just five-and-a-half miles per week and at a pace as casual as about two miles per hour."

Average adult walking speed is approximately three miles an

hour. Your body benefits as much from walking a mile as running a mile — it just takes longer. ("Anywhere is walking distance," quipped comedian Steven Wright, "if you've got the time.") The important thing is that you're not sitting still, which was the focus of a second British survey report, led by Emma Wilmot of the University of Leicester's diabetes research group. Her paper, published in 2012, analyzed 18 studies and the lives of nearly 800,000 participants, and led headline writers to roll out a phrase we're likely to hear a lot more of in the years ahead, one that hearkens back to the work of Richard Doll and Jerry Morris: sitting is the new smoking.

Wilmot's team compared the disease rates of active and inactive adults, and found that people who sit much of the day had a 147 percent greater risk of heart attack or stroke, a 112 percent greater chance of developing diabetes, a 90 percent greater risk of dying from a heart attack and a 49 percent greater risk of premature death. "These are sobering numbers," wrote *Globe and Mail* health reporter André Picard. "The average Canadian adult spends 50 to 70 percent of their daily lives sitting, and roughly 30 percent sleeping. Do the math, and you quickly realize that between sitting in our cars, sitting at our desks at work, sitting in front of the TV, sitting in front of our games consoles, sitting to eat, sitting in school, we hardly move anymore." People who sit most of the day, says Mayo Clinic cardiologist Martha Grogan, have about the same risk of a heart attack as a smoker.

Toronto physician Michael Evans has done the math. Exploring novel ways to speak directly to patients, he made a whiteboard video called *23 and ½ Hours* that has nearly 4.5 million views on YouTube. Evans wanted to tackle the sitting-disease epidemic. He started with a question: even if you are inactive for all but half an hour each day, what's the single most constructive thing you can do for your health in those remaining 30 minutes? Eating more fibre, oral hygiene, regular check-ups — there are many options. But the biggest return on investment, he decided, comes from exercise. Mostly, to be practical, from walking.

That's not a message one hears frequently in our siloed medical system, or from the commercial industries that have developed around obesity, diabetes and heart disease, with the quest for cures often driven by studies financed by pharmaceutical companies. Moreover, funders who donate millions of dollars to hospitals want to buy "fancy new machines," says Evans, not support workaday initiatives to get people moving. "I would do a walking intervention before anything else. Programs that get people active give you more bang for your buck.

"I want to start a movement," he adds. "How can we make our days harder? We need to create a Ministry of Habit."

The medical system is "woefully out of touch," agrees Halifax psychologist Michael Vallis, a professor at Dalhousie University and head of the Orwellian-sounding Behaviour Change Institute (BCI), which teaches health-care providers how to alter their patients' conduct. "It's geared toward acute problems, but lifestyle diseases are overwhelming the system." So many people will be so sick, hospitals and health-care workers won't be able to keep up, and governments won't be able to handle the bills. Forget peak oil — peak Medicare might cripple us first.

Globally, the number of overweight and obese people soared from 857 million to 2.1 billion between 1980 and 2013, according to an article in the *Lancet*. The study, which looked at data from 188 countries, recorded a 28 percent increase among adults and a 47 percent increase in children. Numbers rose in both developed and developing nations. The global economic downturn was a factor. Tough times make people choose food based on price, not nutritional quality, says the Organisation for Economic Co-operation and Development. As unemployment spiked in the U.S. in 2008 and 2009, the consumption of fruits and vegetables declined.

The BCI is focused on healthy eating, physical activity and managing the stresses and strains of daily life. Changing our habits around these core activities is extremely difficult. Often, we are prisoners of the patterns we establish, or the patterns circumstances impose. For years, says Vallis, doctors have said "move more" to sedentary people. Some go so far as to write prescriptions instructing patients to go for a hike. But this approach, like telling smokers to butt out, has limited effectiveness. "This is a complicated problem," says Vallis, "that requires a complicated solution."

When Stanley Vollant holds clinics in Pessamit and other Aboriginal villages, patients often ask him for pills or an operation to remedy their ailments. Regardless of the problem, they don't want to put in the effort themselves. For many, the chasm between who we are and who we want to become is wide, and a reimagined future can feel out of reach. Which is why Vollant says, "You always have to concentrate on the next step, the next hill you're going to climb."

He tells me this as we pull our sleds up a slope on a snow-covered logging road on day three of the expedition. By myself most of yesterday on a 14-mile-long snowmobile trail in the bush, several times I wished I was back home. In the sun, resting briefly, sipping from a thermos of tea, I heard chickadees and spotted fox tracks, and was content. But then the clouds and wind returned. I was tired, cold, alone. So today I hustle to catch up to Vollant.

"Where are we camping tonight?" I ask, uneasy about our first stop without cabins.

Between the road and a small lake, he tells me, a site scouted by Fortin.

"Do you need a permit?"

"Why would we need a permit?" he says, stopping for a swig of water and a bite of moose jerky. "It's our land."

As befits a man with feet in two worlds, Vollant wears Merino wool and Gore-Tex layers under a hand-stitched jacket made from canvas, a technological revolution for the Innu when it was introduced by Europeans in the 1850s. It allowed them to travel light. His gear, wrapped under a blue tarp on a wooden toboggan like the one his grandfather used on hunting trips, includes the bulging red knapsack. Inside are bandages, sterile scissors, cortisone, tensor wraps, moleskin. He lances blisters during morning bush clinics and dispenses Motrin in the middle of the road. Stretching, meditation and traditional knowledge will take you only so far. Sometimes you need modern meds to keep moving.

Vollant did not want to become a doctor. He was going to be a hunter and fisherman like his grandfather, Xavier. Born in Quebec City in 1965, Vollant was put up for adoption by his young single mother, Clarisse, who had been sexually abused at residential school and smothered the pain with alcohol. Xavier got an advance from the Hudson's Bay Company for the next season's furs, flew to the provincial capital and brought four-day-old Stanley back to Pessamit, at the time a village of about 1,500. His mother visited about once a month until she died, too young, on the streets of Montreal. Vollant fished for salmon with his grandfather all summer and hunted for caribou, moose and other game in the fall, sleeping in prospector tents like the ones used by Innu Meshkenu. He went away to high school in Wendake, a reserve in Quebec City, living with a relative but returning home every spring. He wanted to stay in Pessamit, but Xavier, before being killed by a drunk driver in 1982, insisted that his grandson go to university. Afraid not only of blood but also dead bodies, Vollant was set on engineering. He wanted to build dams and roads — "to make a difference in my community." But then, at age 17, he had a bizarre encounter while trying to sneak into a bar with some friends after they had shared a six-pack on the beach.

Phillip, a Pessamit drunk, grabbed Stanley by the hand at the door.

"I want to talk to you," he slurred, spitting in Vollant's face, wobbling unsteadily.

"I don't have time, Phillip."

"I have something very important to tell you."

"Okay, but be quick."

"I heard that you are going to become a doctor."

"No."

"Yes, Stanley."

"No."

"Yes."

To abbreviate the conversation, to catch up with his friends, Vollant agreed.

"I'm so proud of you," said Phillip.

"Okay."

"My parents are proud of you."

"Sure, sure."

"You're going to be the first doctor from the village."

"Sure, okay. Just let me go."

Phillip must have misheard something, Vollant figured the next morning. Still, he couldn't shake the idea, even weeks later, and he applied to the Université de Montréal medical school. Although he fainted before his first dissection session, and fainted again during a clinical immersion in a small Quebec town, his hands were steady and precise from butchering game, and he graduated at age 24, determined to become a surgeon. Only later did he learn that his grandmother, Marianna, had been one of Pessamit's last shamans. She spent time alone with him, and not with other grandchildren, an inheritance he blends seamlessly with Western science.

It's natural for Vollant, one minute, to be talking about serotonin and dopamine, the pleasure chemicals your body secretes when you are active. Alongside endorphins, they diminish pain. The less pain you feel, the less you will reinforce the neural pathways that carry pain signals between the brain and the body. So take Tylenol if you need it, he advises. Then the next minute, he'll morph from medic to mystic and say, "Don't fight with pain. You have to feel some pain to know the meaning of a journey. But if there's too much pain, if you're stuck in the past, the bad memories will keep coming back. It's okay to have memories, to learn from them, but if you're too focused on the pain it's going to get worse."

For some of the walkers — suicidal teenagers, victims of violence, overweight diabetics — this is critical advice. Feel the pain, understand it, let it go. For me, it means accepting that my body and will broke down on a pair of previous multi-day hikes. Prior to the aborted trek to my parents' cottage, I tried to complete Alberta's

200-mile-long Waskahegan Trail in a week. By the second afternoon, my knees and I were done.

Heeding Vollant's counsel, I review the mistakes I made on those two forays into the mild: poor prep, bad boots, heavy loads. Hubris. Haste. I mentally scan my Achilles' heels (post-op right knee: fine; left knee: sore; feet: blister-free; nerves: not bad). Then I will my attention to the rolling road ahead.

Éric Hervieux, 38, who has walked shotgun with Vollant on all but the first trek, is at the front of the pack, as usual. Wearing wrap-around shades and top-of-the-line ski gear, he blazes ahead to the next camp, ensuring there is a warm and comfortable tent ready for his cousin. *Policier* as protector.

Not far behind is Nathalie Dubé, a petite and athletic 47-year-old from Manawan. Dubé started drinking heavily while living with her abusive husband. Now separated and on her second Innu Meshkenu walk, she is sober and 100 pounds lighter. She swapped red meat for fish, nuts and tofu, and walks to and from her job as a receptionist at the elementary school, plus a recreational stroll every evening. Her daily walks average around seven miles, and she looks at least twice that many years younger than her age. "I realized that life is simple," Dubé would tell me, through a translator, a few days later. "I realized that life is beautiful."

Alexandra Awashish, 38, a former band council adviser from Wemotaci, is near the back of the group. She has four kids and lives on social assistance. Her physique is far from sporty. Her feet hurt, her body aches, each hill is a mountain, but in her head, Awashish says, "everything is going into the right place." She wears a Superman cape when she walks and plans to run for chief.

We know that walking can help us live longer, yet we're only starting to understand that where we walk also makes a difference. Roughly 80 percent of Americans live in urban areas with at least 2,500 people, nearly 60 percent in cities of 200,000 or more. One hundred years ago the urban-rural split was 50-50. The numbers are comparable in

Canada. Globally, half of the population had become urban by 2008, a leap from 10 percent a century ago. Densely inhabited cities — walkable cities — are one way to reduce our carbon footprint, and to help us get to know our neighbours. (I'll address these subjects in subsequent chapters.) But beyond exercise, there are other physical benefits associated with getting out of town for a walk. And though the research of Japanese physiological anthropologist Yoshifumi Miyazaki is preliminary, he is doing the same thing as Jerry Morris: trying to substantiate a link that's hidden in plain sight.

Miyazaki, vice-director of the Centre for Environment, Health and Field Sciences at Chiba University, east of Tokyo, is the world's leading expert on "forest bathing." *Shinrin-yoku*, a term introduced by Japan's Ministry of Agriculture, Forestry and Fisheries in 1982, is said to be able to do everything from lowering stress and blood pressure to preventing cancer. These benefits are partially attributed to the presence of phytoncides — the essential-oil-like scents swirling around trees, anti-microbial volatile organic compounds emitted to protect against rotting and insects. Scientists have been looking into their potential medicinal properties since the 1990s. One Japanese study found that mice kept in a fragrant environment enriched with a phytoncide called α-pinene showed reduced melanoma growth.

There are 48 official forest-therapy routes in Japan, and *shinrin-yoku* research has spread to South Korea and Finland, where nascent forest-therapy centres are spending hundreds of thousands of dollars on trails and testing. Miyazaki and his colleagues use hormone analysis, brain imaging and simple measures such as pulse rate and blood-pressure readings to study what happens at a molecular level while people walk in the woods and when they stop. Comparing forest walks with urban walks among more than 600 subjects in his seminal study, Miyazaki concluded that nature yields "a 12.4 percent decrease in the stress hormone cortisol, a seven percent decrease in sympathetic nerve activity, a 1.4 percent decrease in blood pressure, and a 5.8 percent decrease in heart rate." The sympathetic nervous system activates our "fight or flight" response (more on this next chapter). The drop in cortisol levels is significant because cortisol is released as a reaction to stress, and because it inhibits the functioning of our immune system. *Shinrin-yoku*, says Miyazaki, is an "effective and beneficial treatment for people of all ages and backgrounds."

One of his collaborators, Qing Li, an immunologist at Tokyo's Nippon Medical School, is focused on the impact of forest bathing on our natural killer, or NK, cells. These cells attack tumours and help contain bacterial and viral infections. Middle-aged Japanese businessmen who went into the forest for walks experienced NK cell count increases of 40 percent, Li found in one experiment. A month after the trip, levels were still up 15 percent. There was no change among control-group subjects who walked on city streets, although a suburban park will provide an NK boost. In another experiment, Li exposed people to vaporized stem oil from the Hinoki cypress tree in hotel rooms, spurring a 20 percent increase in NK cell counts after three nights compared to the control group. "It's like a miracle drug," he said to *Outside* magazine writer Florence Williams.

But perhaps we shouldn't be surprised. After all, we have lived in a natural environment for 99.99 percent of the past 5 million years, Miyazaki and his team wrote in the *Journal of Physiological Anthropology*: "All human physiological functions have evolved in and adapted to the natural environment . . . the physiological functions of the human are made for the forest."

Li considers forest bathing a preventative medicine, an alternative therapy that encourages relaxation and stress reduction as a way to lower the risk of certain diseases, including cancer. Its tenets are more accepted in Japan than in North America. But things are shifting on this side of the Pacific, and the research being done by Miyazaki, Li and their peers is essential, "a Rosetta stone," naturopathic physician Alan C. Logan, the co-author of *Your Brain on Nature*, said to Williams. "We have to validate the ideas scientifically . . . or we're still stuck at Walden Pond."

Back in Quebec's boreal forest, the barometer is falling. It's night five of the walk, and a storm is coming.

Twice a day, after breakfast and before supper, we form a circle and hold hands. There are prayers, technical briefings, and then, finally, Vollant speaks. "We are bonding," he says each time, "like a big family."

Coming into this trek, I had never sung "Kumbaya." Never went to summer camp. Never said grace. Never gave props to the Creator. Last time I was in a synagogue, it was for a classmate's bar mitzvah, nearly 30 years ago. I was not called to that bar. Spirituality has never been a ritualized practice for me. But here in an earthy temple, gloved fingers entwined with those of a pair of middle-aged women one day, two teenaged boys the next, I have felt it: the kinship of a shared journey. *"Il n'y a pas de culture sans culte,"* Sauvé, who shares my secularism, tells me, quoting French-Canadian writer Jean-Paul Desbiens. There is no culture without cult.

In the 1960s, American psychologist Bruce Tuckman mapped out four stages of group development: forming, storming, norming and performing. We are hitting stage two, and at this evening's circle Vollant calls us out sternly. There's been some bickering among the logisticians, and many of us, including a certain branch schlepper, are not lending a hand as quickly as before. It is taking too long to set up and tear down camp, and wet snow has been falling all day, again, which has made the firewood and tents (and walkers) soggy. Last winter's Innu Meshkenu expedition to Manawan almost broke apart on the fifth day, says Vollant, his voice rising. "You're tired of yourself, and we're tired of each other," he says. "But remember: we are one big family."

Yes, take care of your own needs, but do not rest until everyone else is warm and comfortable. That is how Aboriginal Canadians — all Canadians — used to live. And that is why his grandfather would be rolling over in his grave if he saw how greed and apathy had supplanted the ethos of sharing and resilience among his people today.

"Your toboggan is an important symbol!" thunders Vollant, a preacher on the pulpit. He wants walkers to stop asking logisticians to shuttle their sleds. "Your ancestors pulled 200 pounds in their toboggans. Without them, they would have died. Even if you only carry your water bottle in your sled, take it! We are proud people. We don't want snowmobilers passing by and saying, 'Look at those Indians. They're letting machines do their work.'"

The trouble is, as psychologist Michael Vallis points out, we are hardwired to let machines do our heavy lifting. Western society has "advanced" to the point where the brain's operating system does not serve our best interests. To successfully adapt to our largely urban environment, we need to override three of the basic rules that govern our behaviour. To save calories, we are programmed to choose the path of least resistance. This made sense when we were struggling to survive on the savannah. Today, it's the reason we stand still on escalators, park close to the doors at the mall and purchase the iRobot Roomba 880 to vacuum our floors. Second, we are prisoners of the pleasure principle: avoid pain, seek pleasure. Our choices used to be "run or get eaten by a bear" and "eat some berries or starve." Now we can sit on the La-Z-Boy gorging on jelly doughnuts without fear of being attacked by so much as a mosquito. Finally, we go for instant gratification. We watch TV while shovelling in potato chips, instead of asking, "How will I feel tomorrow if I take a walk today?"

Vallis and his colleagues at the Behaviour Change Institute equip health-care workers with knowledge and techniques they can use to encourage people to get fit and eat healthy — for example, helping people develop "distress tolerance," so they can suck it up during the demoralizing early stages of an exercise regime. Simple measures, like getting off the bus a few stops early, or taking the stairs instead of the escalator, can be effective. Clients in his obesity program get passes for a parking lot one kilometre away from the institute. But the goal is to make these *committed* behaviours, so we opt to walk regardless of the weather and our moods. The American Heart Association recommends 30 minutes of brisk walking five days a week, and notes that walking has the lowest dropout rate of any physical activity. And though the gains are modest, the health benefits of inching from sedentary to slightly active are more pronounced than the jump from average to extreme athlete. Fat but fit people will live longer than those who are average weight but inactive, and the rate of return on exercise diminishes after about an hour a day. Unfortunately, these types of habits can take at least two years to find purchase, an eternity for policy-makers governed by the bottom line and politicians who can't see beyond the next election.

Like Dr. Michael Evans, Vallis wants to address more than the symptoms of sitting disease. In his view, we need to reimagine the built environment (instead of widening roads, improve sidewalks) and remove the agricultural subsidies that support the proliferation of high-fructose corn syrup, which lights up the limbic system like cocaine. Less screen time wouldn't hurt, especially because the media culture that has made "Go big or go home" a mantra is partially to blame. Television shows such as *The Biggest Loser*, fad and crash diets and a running craze in which ultra-marathons are the new marathons set people up for failure. "We need to promote doable and sustainable activities," says Vallis. "Walking is not jockish. It speaks to a huge percentage of the population. Slow and steady wins the race."

Amid this shift in medical thinking, however, University of Toronto kinesiology professor and health communication specialist Margaret MacNeill issues a cautionary note. Arthritic knees respond well to a strict workout schedule; post–heart attack exercise programs are curative. "But if you medicalize exercise, you make it a dose," she says, "full of little formulas, measures you might not achieve."

Medicalization, a concept developed by sociologist Irving Zola in the 1970s, is the process by which human situations come to be regarded as medical conditions, as problems that require treatment. For instance, pregnancy. There are benefits to this process, which is rooted in scientific knowledge. The Canada Fitness Test — six standardized activities all grade-school students in the country were forced to do in the 1970s and 1980s, including the painful flexed arm hang, earning excellence, gold, silver or bronze awards, or lowly participant badges — is an example of medicalization applied to exercise. The program encouraged physical health, but the delivery method stigmatized tens of thousands of children (including yours truly, a chubby eight-year-old), and reinforced a singular image of the body and its possibilities. "With medicalization, we narrowly construct the problem and narrowly search for solutions," says MacNeill. "We lose touch with what physical activity should be: social and fun. You know the phrase 'exercise is medicine'? It can be, but not for everybody.

"Walking can't solve all our problems, but I think it's our best possibility right now. It's more than exercise. It is life."

After Vollant's sermon, the mood in camp is dour, so I hide away by sequestering Napech for an interview in the cook tent. Sitting on an overturned plastic bucket, he is quiet after each of my questions: eyes closed, sometimes nodding, the occasional sigh. "I'm here to spend time in nature, with the children," he says finally, through a translator. "It makes me feel younger." More silence. Then, when I wonder whether he is dozing off, he says, "Life is like an arrow. You have the tip, the shaft, the feathers. The tip represents the youth, the shaft represents the adults, the feathers are the elders. The arrow is balanced when all of the parts come together. That's why it flies so well."

Even though we're deep in the forest, my weary brain churns as I digest this simile.

Next, Napech tells me he's a medicine man, so I complain that I have a sore neck from sleeping on the ground.

"Take off your jacket," he instructs.

He massages my neck, then places a hand on both sides of my chin and lifts my head firmly, a jarring chiropractic adjustment.

Then he tells me not to think about the pain.

Rolling my shoulders, I retreat to my little family's tent, where Vollant informs me that we'll be staying up in shifts to keep the wet wood burning and avoid getting smoked out. "If I die before I wake," he says, rolling into his sleeping bag, "pray the Lord my soul to take."

"The Bible?" I ask.

"No, Metallica. 'Enter Sandman.' I'm a big heavy-metal guy."

Sauvé takes the first watch, waking me at midnight. I stoke the stove, then slip outside to pee. The night is still, clear. A row of 10 smoking chimneys. Snoring muffled by canvas. Half a dozen snow-mobiles are parked on the logging road. It resembles a blockade. We are following a route the Innu traditionally travelled to recruit Atikamekw and other allies for their battles against the English, but Vollant calls this a mission of peace.

After his pep talk, and a smoky night, and a fraternal reprimand from my tent-mates, the 5 a.m. reveille sparks a resilient energy. Giant steel pots of water are boiled on propane burners for coffee, tea and oatmeal. A table outside the cook tent is decked with bags of bagels and packets of peanut butter. There are slabs of ham and a heaping bowl of scrambled eggs. (Fortin's shopping list included 90 pounds of cheese, 35 pounds of jerky and 35 pounds of nuts.) After eating and packing a lunch, I help skewer the branches we used as bedding onto sticks, which will be put into aluminum boats and towed behind snowmobiles to the next site, along with leftover firewood and the birch poles used to frame the tents. Soon, flattened rectangles of snow and a pile of smoking stoves are all that remain of camp.

This morning's circle is cheerful, and I cover two dozen kilo-metres like an arrow, pulling my sled the entire distance, except on long, steep descents, where I unbuckle my waist belt, hop on top and slide down at GPS-logged speeds topping 25 miles an hour, whooping wildly.

I started the journey as a mildly neurotic urban professional, as a journalist immersed in a story, but as the days beat on, lines blur. I leave Fleischman in its stuff sack, join men hunting partridge and foraging for wood and crack jokes in halting French, at one point impersonating Hervieux using his police badge to confiscate a bucket of fried chicken: *"Venir avec moi, poulet frit!"* I'm the one initiating bear hugs now.

Tonight's destination is the community hall in the village of Lac-Saint-Paul, where there will be a pay phone for calling home, a dépanneur for chocolate and a dry floor for us to sleep on — all crammed together, a jumble of bodies, as if in an emergency shelter. A week ago, such a scenario would have sent me running, but ascending another snowy hill, undeterred by what might be around the corner, I grasp, at last, that walking is a way to push toward change at a sustainable pace, to leave one comfort zone and begin to forge another.

Napech may glide down hills on his pulk, but he's hardier than most elders. Snow and ice limit mobility in our cities, especially among seniors and people with disabling illnesses and injuries. For some, even dry city sidewalks and climate-controlled interiors are difficult to navigate. So a few months after Innu Meshkenu, I buttoned up a borrowed parka and stepped into a simulated winter environment four storeys beneath the streets of downtown Toronto to see how cutting-edge science is helping keep people active.

It is 20° Fahrenheit inside WinterLab, a 20-by-18-foot pod with an ice floor and fans that can generate winds of 20 miles an hour. Jennifer Hsu, a PhD student studying biomedical engineering, tightens my construction safety harness and clips me into an overhead line. I am wearing a pair of boots with flat treadless soles. They are made by a South Korean company called JStep using a proprietary rubber compound that has impressive slip resistance. (The J stands for Jesus. The company's logo was modelled after the green basilisk lizard, also known as the Jesus Christ lizard, for its ability to dart across water.)

When most researchers test the frictional properties of footwear, they use a machine that drags the sole over a stainless-steel surface sprayed with glycerol. Here, Hsu has a real person, plus a bucket of water and a cooler full of snow, which she can spread on the ice. WinterLab can also be lifted onto a hydraulic motion platform and titled up to 23 degrees, and test subjects can be shaken with a sudden acceleration of up to 26 feet/second squared to assess how they (and their boots) respond to slips and slides. "What we're trying to understand," says Hsu, "is how people actually walk in winter conditions."

WinterLab is one of three pods at the Toronto Rehabilitation Institute's $36 million Challenging Environment Assessment Laboratory, the flagship of the institute's iDAPT (Intelligent Design for Adaptation, Participation and Technology) Centre. CEAL opened in 2011, marshalling together the experience and interests of nearly 100 scientists and twice as many grad students. The other two pods are StreetLab, which uses a 270-degree curved screen, surround-sound system and treadmill to simulate the streetscape above, allowing researchers to study how pedestrians respond to the sights, noises and physical sensations of the city, including tiny details, like the slight rumbling underfoot when a streetcar passes; and StairLab, which researchers can outfit with staircases or ramps of varying geometries, with or without handrails, to test balance and recovery and help devise safe configurations. Reflective markers worn on clothing and shoes, motion-capture sensors on the walls of the pods, and force plates underfoot measure every grip, step and stumble, providing an extremely comprehensive account of why we move the way we do, and what design changes can help keep us upright.

"We've been doing research on human balance and fall prevention in my labs for about 30 years," says Toronto Rehab's head of research, Geoff Fernie, a bioengineer and University of Toronto surgery professor, "and honestly, it hasn't had a lot of impact when you compare it with introducing seat belts and reducing tobacco use. The emphasis we're now placing on the environment is probably the way to go. That's where the low-hanging fruit is. We may not be able to change the way people behave, but we sure as hell can make stairs and intersections safer."

A visit to CEAL is like a trip to Q Branch, the mad-scientist lair where James Bond's spy gadgets are created (albeit with no pens that shoot explosive darts). In the elevator ride down to the cavernous basement facility, a guy in a white lab coat showed me a prototype sleep-apnea device, a lightweight and flexible V-shaped wireless unit that's worn over the nose and mouth at home to diagnose the breathing disorder. Eighty-five percent of all cases of sleep apnea go undetected, it is estimated, which leads to billions of dollars in medical costs in the United States every year (e.g., drowsy people crashing their cars on the way to work in the morning).

The price we pay for falling is equally staggering. In Canada, the social and health-care cost of accidents on stairs alone is estimated at $8.8 billion a year. Like the rising price tag associated with medical treatment for the country's growing Aboriginal population, falls are becoming more of a problem as the continent's population ages. From 1997 to 2009, the rate of hospitalization from injuries on home stairs in the U.S. increased an average of 6 percent each year. Seniors are the most likely to get hurt this way. One in three people over 65 falls every year in Canada, half of them more than once, and 40 percent of serious falls result in hip fractures. These accidents can precipitate a downward spiral. Inactivity leads to ill health, which leads to isolation, fear and more inactivity. "Twenty percent of all injury-related deaths among seniors can be traced back to a fall," reports the Public Health Agency of Canada. One in five older adults who suffer hip fractures will die within 12 months of their injury. "If we don't do something," says Fernie, "we're going to have to build hospitals that don't do anything but fix hips."

Staircases are an important front for CEAL, and a victory may be near. After wiping out a few times in WinterLab — conventional chunky treads appear to work better than JStep soles when there is water or snow atop the ice — I meet StairLab's lead researcher, post-doctoral fellow Alison Novak. Canada's building code currently calls for private dwellings to have steps with at most an eight-inch vertical riser and at least an 8.25-inch horizontal run. Safety researchers have been proposing longer step runs for two decades, but the building industry is resistant to change. "Their primary argument," says Novak, "is cost." Longer steps require more material and a larger footprint for staircases in new homes. Thousands of blueprints would have to be sent back to the drawing board.

Novak used StairLab to get a better understanding of foot trajectory and balance control among young adults (aged 18 to 35) and healthy older adults (65 plus) on staircases with runs that spanned 8 to 14 inches at one-inch intervals. Future studies will look at people with disabilities; building codes are designed around the general population. Her results, obtained by shaking the pod on the motion platform to analyze when and how people fell, determined that increasing the minimum length of residential steps to 10 inches will decrease falls by a factor of four. Two years of evidence generated by Novak was submitted to the National Building Code's Joint Task Group on Step Dimensions, which recommended a change during one of its regular review cycles. The week I visited CEAL, in autumn 2013, she went to Montreal to attend a meeting of the Standing Committee on Housing and Small Buildings, where members voted unanimously to increase minimum run length to 10 inches. This change became law in 2015, with the regulators declaring that the new dimensions "could reduce fall incidences by up to 64 percent."

At the same time as she works to help prevent such trauma, Novak and Vicki Komisar, a PhD student whose thesis will investigate the optimal height of handrails on staircases and ramps, are developing new ways to *make* people fall. Novak gives me a pair of running shoes with reflective markers and another safety harness, and, like astronauts about to blast off, we take the elevator up one storey to CEAL mission control. We walk over a bridge and through a metal door into the pod that usually houses StairLab. Today, its surface is a flat, rectangular platform of eight four-foot-squared force plates. Novak clips me into the overhead line, then straps herself into a jump seat with a three-point belt. The pod begins to tilt on the motion platform, reaching a 10-degree slope. Watching on a monitor and communicating with us from the control room via a two-way radio, Komisar instructs me to begin counting down from 100 in threes and to walk back and forth on the platform. After a few seconds, the pod shakes, but I only stumble slightly. Following a few more rounds, walking back and forth and counting to myself until getting jostled unexpectedly, I change into a pair of shoes with cotton covering the soles. These have very little slip resistance, and when the pod shakes, only the harness prevents me from slamming into the wall. Had there been a handrail, I would have grabbed it. Novak and Komisar compare notes. This appears to be an effective way to simulate falling.

Research like this is painstaking. But it's faster than frame-by-frame analysis of acetate film, as their predecessors once did. And to get solutions quickly from the lab to the real world, Fernie says, "you have to replicate the real world as well as possible."

Fernie was in a wheelchair when I toured CEAL. He had hurt his back lifting snow tires in his garage. After returning to work, being bumped around in crowded elevators and looking colleagues in the belly while in conversation, he got a glimpse of life with limited mobility. "You become dependent on other people. Your life changes if you can't get around," he says. "If we don't do something to help people continue to be mobile, to get the exercise they need, so their cardiovascular fitness is there, so they're happy and interactive, if we don't do that, their lives will change for the worse. It's fundamental."

At around noon on February 27, 1992, Amanda Boxtel, an Australian transplanted to Colorado, rode the chairlift to the top of the mountain at Snowmass, just down the valley from Aspen. The sporty, blonde 24-year-old was an excellent skier. She chose an intermediate run, and stopped on the flats halfway down to take in the view. A sea of snow-capped peaks stretched to the horizon. When she launched herself forward and continued her descent, Boxtel's ski tips crossed and she did a somersault, landing on her back. A sensation like electricity shot through her legs. Ski patrollers brought her to the base of the mountain and she was airlifted to a hospital in Denver. She had shattered four vertebrae. Two weeks later, a doctor said the words she was dreading: "You will never walk again."

Paralyzed from the waist down and confined to a wheelchair, Boxtel learned how to use a mono-ski. She became a disabled ski instructor, co-founded a charity that provides access to sports and recreational activities for people with disabilities and carried the Olympic torch in 2002. She also took up cycling, rock climbing, paragliding, kite-surfing and scuba diving, and joined the first disabled whitewater rafting trip through the Grand Canyon. Still, she felt a burning need to walk. "I wanted to be able to support myself on my own legs," she says. "It's always been alive in me."

In the first five years after her accident, Boxtel tried everything to regain feeling in and use of her legs: raw-food diets, meditation, acupuncture, shamanistic healing sessions in New Mexico. She pursued every naturopathic methodology she had heard of — drawing the line at shark cartilage injections — as well as conventional cures, including intensive physiotherapy and heavy leg braces. Nothing worked. In 2007, Boxtel decided to try one final experimental treatment. She flew to India, where a doctor at a private hospital injected embryonic stem cells into her spinal cord, a controversial practice. Boxtel received six doses of the cells, and, for the first time in more than 15 years, she began to feel sensations in her legs again. Over time, the feelings grew stronger. She could wriggle her toes. Trace muscle power in her quadriceps, hamstrings and glutes returned. Boxtel could urinate without help from an implanted electronic device, and she could orgasm. All of this only renewed her will to walk.

Turning to technology, she tried an anti-gravity treadmill, zipping into a kayaklike skirt and flailing her legs on a cushion of air. It was like walking, but her body was out of alignment and not weight-bearing. Her heels weren't striking the ground and sending feedback to her brain. "I could swing my legs sloppily, like a drunkard," she says. "It wasn't pretty."

In her dreams, Boxtel saw herself as an avatar, as "Perfect Amanda," encased in some sort of robotic outfit. She wrote to a researcher at Stanford University, asking to participate in a virtual reality experiment. She never heard back. Then she got a phone call from a California company called Berkeley Bionics (now Ekso Bionics). They had a prototype exoskeleton suit and were looking for test pilots. After 18 years of paralysis, with the cameras from National Geographic Television rolling, Boxtel was strapped into the robotic legs. The machine stood her up. It bent her knee. She took a step. Then another. And then one more. That night, she returned to her hotel room and wept.

Wired magazine dubbed the exoskeleton the second most significant gadget of 2010. The iPod was number one.

Three years after that walk, Boxtel is an ambassador for Ekso and owns one of the company's 50-pound EKSO 1.1 units. It has a computer, a gyroscope, two batteries, six joints, four motors and hundreds of sensors. She slides into it from a wheelchair. It encases her legs, the metal shafts akin to one's skeletal structure. The motors are like her muscles; the sensors like nerves. When she begins attempting to take a step, the robot lets her contribute what she can using her own muscles, then powers her through the rest of the motion. Once she shifts her weight correctly, the unit determines that it's time for another step. "I play a central role in my walking," says Boxtel, "but this is the most complex neural prosthetic ever created. It's the fusion of biology and technology."

It also has a name — Tucker, a tribute to her dearly departed golden retriever.

Boxtel and Tucker walk for an hour a day, with a physical therapist nearby to ensure she doesn't fall. The exoskeleton doesn't have a fall-prevention mechanism. It's supposed to be used on flat indoor surfaces, but Boxtel has taken it outside, and she lives in the mountains, where even parking lots have a slope. Machines like the Ekso 1.1 cost between $80,000 and $150,000. It is still a therapeutic device — there are no models on the market for personal use yet. But Boxtel participated in an experiment in Budapest in 2013: a body scan and 3-D printer were used to make custom parts for Tucker. She foresees a day when regenerative medicine and biotech change the landscape for victims of spinal injuries.

Not all wheelchair users share her enthusiasm. When a young man in an exoskeleton kicked a soccer ball during the opening ceremony for the 2014 World Cup, Red Nicholson, a teacher in New Zealand who used to run a blog called Walking Is Overrated, responded to the media frenzy: "Ask any wheelchair user, particularly one who's been in the game awhile, and they'll tell you that they're far too busy living their lives to sit there worrying about whether or not they'll ever walk. I have no more desire to be strapped to a robot than I do to go swimming with great white sharks . . . my life as a wheelchair-user is a very good one."

Still, Boxtel is the type of person who probably would want to swim with sharks. There's a video of one of the first times she walked in an exoskeleton. She is visiting New York City. There she is, jostled by tourists, walking with Tucker on the observation deck of the Empire State Building. "Oh my gosh!" she shrieks. "Twenty years — twenty years of paralysis. Now I get to stand up and look at the view."

Pulks don't glide well on gravel shoulders. After our night on the floor of the community hall in Lac-Saint-Paul, where walkers bought every single piece of fruit in the dépanneur but ignored the beer fridge, we exit the forest and zigzag along a series of rural roads and secondary highways, leaving Atikamekw land and pushing into Anishinabe territory. Fortin's logisticians load our sleds into a cube van, and we average 17 miles a day for five days. The longest walk of the expedition is 22 miles, to the town of Maniwaki, adjacent to the Kitigan Zibi reserve, where we'll rest for two nights before the final week of walking.

Fuelled by rabbit pie and spaghetti with moose sauce, I decide to bust out ahead of Hervieux on the way to our rendezvous point in Maniwaki. It's not a race, but I'm feeling strong. I pack my knapsack strategically, energy bars and water at the ready, and eat and drink without stopping, glancing back over my shoulder periodically until I can no longer see Hervieux. Five hours later, I'm in the parking lot of the Château Logue Hotel.

After everybody arrives, we take a bus to the reserve and walk en masse to the school for another feast. I return the next morning with Vollant, who makes presentations to students of every age, from kindergarten to graduating seniors. As progressively older classes come to the library to listen, he refines his delivery to match their maturity. But he always circles back to two points. Vollant asks the kids what they want to be when they grow up. Hockey player? Teacher? Hunter? Astronaut? He tells them about Dr. Raven Dumont, a girl from Kitigan Zibi who saw him speak when she was a teenager and is now a medical resident in Montreal. "Hopefully at least one of you will become a doctor," he says, "because I'm going to need a very good Aboriginal orthopedic surgeon for my knees after all this walking." Then he shifts into public-service-announcement mode and tells the students to spend more time outside. "On my walks, there is no television, no Nintendo. The only game is cutting wood."

Some of the high school students look bored. They fidget. Vollant becomes more serious. He tells them how the Innu have lost traditional land to flooding from Hydro Québec dams. How his grandfather pushed him to go to university and help his people. Here in the school library, when Vollant talks about the importance of having a dream, he doesn't sound like a shaman. More like Martin Luther King, Jr.

The home stretch of the expedition is elastic. We are fully on Indian time. Each day, we walk until reaching camp, then we work, eat and sleep, and begin anew in the morning, a suspended state of fatigued bliss. I spend an afternoon walking with Devin Petiquay, a 16-year-old from Manawan, a long-haired teen I might have crossed a dark street to avoid in the city. Other than this trip and our gender, we have little in common, yet we share snacks and manage an extended conversation about hockey and hunting, and he teaches me a few Atikamekw words: *nimitsoun* (eat), *misigwam* (toilet), *nimoutan* (walk). Life *is* simple.

Fortin's trailer blows an axle, but it breaks just outside the town of Mont-Laurier, a snowmobile touring mecca that may have more welders per capita, he posits, than anywhere else in Canada. The unit is roadworthy again in a few hours. My sleeping bag catches fire one night, but a tent-mate smells the smoke and wakes me; he has a patch kit and duct tape, and my scare makes for a good story at breakfast. Near the tiny village of Montcerf-Lytton, the proprietor of Fromagerie la Cabriole chases a couple of walkers — and hands them a sack of artisanal chèvre made with port. He had read about the walk in a local newspaper. A stray dog, a dead ringer for the Littlest Hobo, joins the expedition that day, remaining with us throughout the final week. These are random occurrences, of course, but stringing them together, like stones leading across a river, it is hard not to ascribe meaning.

We have permission to travel along one of Quebec's main snowmobile routes for the last four days, through a provincial wildlife reserve, to the Anishinabe village of Rapid Lake. We number fewer at this point; not even Vollant's toenail-removal operations could keep some walkers on their feet. Those of us who continue slow down after the break. There are long rises to climb, and though some rare bright sunshine allows us to strip down to T-shirts, it also makes the snow soggy and the sleds harder to pull.

At one campsite atop a frozen marsh, a damp, dreary evening when the temptation to hole up in my sleeping bag with a book grows strong, I find myself at the woodpile, amid a ring of shining headlamps, where Alexandra Awashish shows me how to rotate a log to find the grain and strike hard with a heavy axe blade at a slight angle. Also, how to say *tabernac* correctly, with the accent on the final syllable. I misfire with the axe a few times — *"TaberNAC!"* — then find the sweet spot and start splitting rounds with one swing. "You," says Super Alex, "would make a good Indian."

There's a towering bonfire in the middle of the circle on our final night together. As semis roar past on the highway beyond the edge of camp, Napech and the other elders recite prayers. Then Leo Dubé, a logistician from Manawan, drums and sings a rousing song, his metronomic strokes and undulating falsetto — "ya hey-ya-hey hey-ya, ya hey-ya-hey hey-ya" — rising above the crackling of dead branches.

Vollant nods to the beat, arms crossed, head down. After the song, he asks everyone to take a turn speaking. I thank the *marcheurs* for sharing their land and culture, for overturning prejudices I had harboured, for helping me learn a few things about myself.

When everyone is finished, Vollant peers around the circle, the firelight reflecting off his yellow parka. "Listen to me," he says quietly. "I'm speaking as a physician. Right now, we feel really good because of the endorphins we've generated. This sense of well-being can last for three or four weeks. But then you can fall into a deep depression. It happens to Olympic athletes, to people who climb Mount Everest. It's normal, not a sign of weakness."

Heads hang, boots kick at the snow. Hours away from our triumphant walk into Rapid Lake, this is not what we want to hear. But most of us are starting to figure out that, on its own, the act of putting one foot in front of the other cannot solve anything. That a circle has no finish line. Our bodies may be stronger, but shadows persist.

When you get home, rest for a couple of days, recommends Vollant. Drink water. Wean yourself off high-carb meals. Talk to people if you feel troubled. Then, when your blisters have healed, keep on walking.

two

MIND

"Right now, we are deciding, without quite meaning to, which evolutionary pathways will remain open and which will forever be closed. No other creature has ever managed this, and it will, unfortunately, be our most enduring legacy."
— *Elizabeth Kolbert,* The Sixth Extinction

"I know of no thought so burdensome that one cannot walk away from it."
— *Søren Kierkegaard*

A gunmetal sky spits warm rain onto Eglinton Street. Truck engines grumble. Brakes hiss and belch. Across the River Clyde from downtown Glasgow, the exhaust-choked thoroughfare parallels the rail corridor that runs south from Central Station and passes beneath the monolithic green girders of the M74 motorway. Lined by dodgy kebab shops, betting dens with broken windows, discount auto mechanics and graffiti-covered concrete walls, this is not a pleasant strip to stroll during the afternoon rush. At several intersections, the sidewalk is hemmed in by waist-high metal barriers, forcing me to detour laterally along cross streets before continuing south.

A solo walk through an unfamiliar swath of urbanity will usually invigorate me, no matter how unappealing the environs or weather.

During the decade that I lived in Edmonton, which has among the most frigid winters of any large city on the planet, and an orderly grid of numbered streets, shifting my commute by a single block would reveal small wonders. The high-pitched song of snow under boot at -35° Fahrenheit. A magpie stencilled onto a letterbox, its speech bubble urging passersby to listen. Candles flickering inside cylinders made of ice.

I have vivid memories of walking from my sister-in-law's house in the extreme northeast corner of Calgary, whose sprawling footprint is the size of Chicago, to a strip-mall bistro in the inner burbs, cutting through eerily empty subdivisions and industrial parks that were still under construction, sleeping bulldozers and stacks of rebar casting skeletal shadows in the lamp-lit darkness. The price of oil was soaring. Alberta had one of the fastest-growing gross domestic products on the planet. People were moving to the province from around the world. By walking through the edgelands, I got an intimate look at the seams beneath the boom.

That same year, I spent a week in Fort McMurray, the heart of Canada's tar sands, camping on the fringe of the city and walking to downtown appointments along arterial roads with vehicles whizzing past at highway speed. "Be careful," the young drywallers living year-round at the next site had warned. "Nobody walks around here." I surveyed the litter in the ditches (Tim Hortons cups, cans of Black Horse beer from Newfoundland, lottery tickets) and counted pickup trucks. It was fascinating. A new frontier.

Today, however, after spending the afternoon on foot in Glasgow, I'm feeling weary and, well, *sad*. Which is an appropriate starting point, because I have come to the most unhealthy city in the United Kingdom to find out whether walking can really help make people more happy.

Scotland has the lowest life expectancy in Western Europe, and Glaswegians meet their makers well before the British average: men at age 72.6, versus 78.9, and women at 78.5, versus 82.7. Researchers blame this mortality gap on a mysterious phenomenon known as "the

Glasgow effect." In other words, they don't have a good explanation. Poverty, poor diet, violence, smoking and substance abuse all play a role, as is the case in Aboriginal Canada. But even when compared to similar post-industrial cities, such as Liverpool and Manchester, Glasgow is hurting; its inhabitants are 30 percent more likely to die young. Drugs, alcohol, suicide and crime are behind 60 percent of these deaths. And all this pain has triggered a mental-health problem as well.

The Scottish Health Survey's 2010 examination of the Glasgow effect, a comprehensive analysis that controlled for socio-economic, behavioural, biological and other mitigating factors, found that residents had a 92 percent greater risk of anxiety than people living elsewhere in the country. They also had significantly higher scores on the General Health Questionnaire — an indicator of "possible psychiatric disorder."

There are many plausible, interrelated reasons for the differences between Glaswegians and their Liverpudlian and Mancunian cousins, a quartet of researchers concluded in a paper they wrote for the Glasgow Centre for Population Health. To be precise, they came up with 17 hypotheses, ranging from genetic and cultural scenarios to the gloomy weather and the lingering impacts of a politically motivated attack instigated by Margaret Thatcher. At least three dozen public programs have been launched to help heal the city. Beyond smoking bans and a minimum-price-per-unit-of-alcohol campaign, police officers are stationed at some schools, and dentists and veterinarians are trained to watch for signs of domestic abuse. "We took the attitude that [the problem is] so big and so complex, it doesn't make any difference where you start," one senior police officer told the *Guardian*. "Just make a bloody start."

I'm plodding along Eglinton's gritty streetscape, past shuttered grocery stores and fences topped with razor wire, to meet some people who have taken this message to heart: members of a health-walk program that was created to give locals a badly needed boost.

My day began on a much more bucolic note. I woke up 80 miles south of Glasgow in an 18th-century country inn. The Ken Bridge, named after the adjacent five-arch granite bridge over the Water of Ken, is on the old road between Ireland and Edinburgh. Built to provide food, drink and shelter for stagecoach travellers, it did so admirably for me for two days. I was in the area to interview a man who lives in the nearby village of New Galloway, a geographer who had hiked the length of Ireland and Scotland. When we weren't walking and talking together, I sipped pints of ale in the Ken Bridge's cozy wood-panelled pub and roamed the path between the inn and the village, letting the birdsong wash over me while standing chest-deep in the fen and willow scrub of a nature reserve.

Upon returning to the pub after one such ramble, I asked if it was safe to swim in the river.

"Aye, you can," nodded Willie, the hotel's maintenance man, "but you've got to watch out for sharks."

"In this place," added a bearded bear of a man, who turned out to be a distinguished Scottish historian named Ted Cowan, sitting on his regular stool at the end of the row, "most of the sharks are at the bar."

"No, really, it's fine," chimed in the Ken Bridge's owner, Dave Paterson. "The last person who swam here was a Buddhist monk from Holland."

"Did he come back?"

"She did. You'll be following good footsteps."

I walked upriver from the bridge, stripped naked on a stony beach and waded into the warm green water, lazing in a deep pool until a lorry rumbled by and honked.

The next morning, I stood beside the highway that ran past the inn and held up my thumb. "Nobody hitchhikes here," I had been cautioned at the bar. Ten minutes later, a van eased onto the shoulder, and a balding middle-aged man shoved some gear aside to clear off the passenger seat. We hit construction, and Neil Stout, a picture-framing machine repairman on his way to a job in

Glasgow, got an earful from his GPS when he was forced to divert off the pre-programmed direct route. "It's a helpful device," he said, pressing buttons forcefully with his index finger, unsure which town we were in or which road we were on, "but you lose the identity of where you are. It's astonishing how fast the human race is losing all these skills."

As we rolled past fields dotted with hay bales and 17th-century tower houses, our conversation flitted from subject to subject but never waned, as is often the case in the covenant struck between hitchhiker and driver. When I said I was here to learn more about British walking culture, Stout told me about the time an old rugby neck injury flared up and he thought he might die. Doctors had to perform an emergency cervical laminectomy. Stout had three goals before the operation: he wanted to walk out of the hospital; to get strong enough to climb Scafell Pike, the highest mountain in England; and to record an album. The first two things happened, he said. Then he plugged his iPod into the van's stereo. A bluesy, acoustic track began, raspy lyrics sung by a guy who sounded like Eric Clapton. Stout's album is called *Humble*. The song: "Heaven." We listened in silence.

He dropped me off in central Glasgow, a dozen blocks from my hotel, a Euro-cool boutique chain targeted at the "smart new breed of international traveller . . . the type who crosses continents the way others cross streets," although the "ambassador" who checked me in admitted he was Glaswegian — "Aye, I'm a local for my sins." I didn't feel hip enough to hang out in the lounge amid the sleek, Danish modern furniture (and sleek, modern, possibly Danish guests). Instead, I put on my boots and crossed the street.

The name Glasgow is derived from a Gaelic word that means "dear, green place." Despite the health statistics and the drizzle, the city was far from bleak on a mild summer afternoon. There was a lively pedestrian mall near my hotel, and I ambled through packs of umbrella-toting families along an attractive waterfront promenade on the Clyde. Even the scrap iron and fibreglass riverside statue of

Spanish Civil War hero Dolores Ibárruri, both fists raised defiantly skyward, seemed to speak to walking. "Better to die on your feet," read the inscription, "than live forever on your knees."

When the rain intensified, I ducked into the palatial Kelvingrove Art Gallery and Museum, and found exhibits on industrialization and mental health on display in adjacent rooms. On a fine Sunday morning in early 1765, a 29-year-old mathematical instrument maker named James Watt went for a walk in Glasgow Green, less than a mile from Eglinton Street. For months, he had been struggling with an engineering puzzle: how could he design a full-sized engine with cylinders that didn't have to be cooled after every stroke? Near the wash house where women laundered their linens before spreading them on the grass to dry, inspiration struck: a separate condenser vessel for the steam. "I had not walked farther than the golf house," Watt said later, "when the whole thing was arranged in my mind." The next day — because it was forbidden to tinker in his lab on the Sabbath — he successfully built and tested the first model of the "modern" steam engine.

Watt's invention sent the Industrial Revolution into overdrive. It has been pinpointed by American ecologist Eugene Stoermer and Nobel Prize–winning Dutch atmospheric chemist Paul Crutzen as the start of the Anthropocene — our current geological era, distinct from times past because human activities are now having a significant impact on the earth's ecosystems.

The shock waves from Watt's eureka moment radiated globally, and Glasgow quickly grew to be Scotland's largest city. Perhaps not coincidentally, it also became the site of Britain's first purpose-built mental asylum, which opened in 1814: "a house," according to the Kelvingrove's interpretive panel, "with proper keepers adapted to the situation of those diseased in their minds." By 1900, three more sanatoriums had been built on country estates on the outskirts of town. This approach evolved. Out-of-the-way stowage asylums were replaced by hospitals focused on cures, and since the 1990s the emphasis has been on care in the community.

As I exit the museum, cross the Clyde and begin my walk along Eglinton, I can't stop thinking about connections between the two exhibits. Industrial manufacturing flourished but now sputters in Scotland, leaving a strewn field of crumbling factories, unemployment and sorrow, the seeping vapours that fuel the Glasgow effect.

Though tempted to retreat to the bosom of free, on-demand movies in my sleek hotel room, I continue south and enter the lobby of the New Victoria Hospital, where members of the walking group are meeting at 6 p.m. Seven women and two men, all wearing sensible shoes, sit on plastic chairs outside the cafeteria. Walk Glasgow coordinator Heather Macleod, 30-something with curly blond hair and a clipboard, introduces the regulars and explains the routine while we wait for stragglers. Funded by a non-profit called Paths for All and Scotland's National Heath Service, the volunteer-led walks, which are offered in all corners of the city, year round, last about an hour. These free outings encourage people to be active and social. They're intended to promote a general sense of well-being, particularly in parts of Glasgow where health inequalities are most pronounced. "Getting out in a group," Macleod says, "you become part of a new community. It's not the physical benefits that keep walkers coming out. It's the people they meet."

"Remember the golden rule," Val Kennedy, this evening's leader, a stout woman with grey hair and thick glasses, announces as we leave the hospital. "Walk and talk. Of course, you cannae stop people in Glasgow from chattin'."

We cross a busy road and enter Queen's Park, 150 acres of lawns, thickets and sports fields developed in the late 19th century, a Victorian response to the proliferation of crowded tenements. Mindful of Kennedy's directive, I fall into step beside 38-year-old Ian McVicar. A large man with broad shoulders and a buzz cut, McVicar spent 18 years working in a timber yard, feeding the cutting machines and checking wood quality. "Ah was a saw-yer," he says in a thick Glaswegian brogue, sliding his thick arm and flattened hand back and forth horizontally, as if slicing through a two-by-four. "Like Tom Saw-yer." After his shift, he would go home and watch football on television. McVicar had been diagnosed with schizophrenia as a teenager, and the routine gave him structure. When he was medically retired from the timber yard two years ago, he fell into a deep depression. Then he started walking. "Ah hae ne'er dain anythin' loch thes afair," he says. "Ah hae come out of mah sheel."

McVicar, who now does three or four different health walks every week, has lost a stone and a half (about 20 pounds) since getting off the couch. He sleeps better. And he has enrolled in college-level reading and writing courses, hoping to eventually qualify for a job in the admin sector. McVicar is meeting new people, and never feels any animosity: "Afair, ah did nae caur abit anythin'. Ah am lookin' at life deefrant noo."

Buoyed by this tête-à-tête, I mingle. Red-haired Betty Ferry, 59, says she has a bad back and arthritic knees. Because of her weight and age, she's not a good candidate for knee surgery. She's tired after these walks, but, as with McVicar, it's the kind of tired that leads to a clear mind and a good sleep. Ferry has twin daughters, as do I, and we trade stories as we leave the park and enter a neighbourhood of sandstone merchant houses long ago divided into flats.

Banding into small clusters on the narrow sidewalk, Ferry and I are joined by Kennedy, her sister. Kennedy suffers from seasonal affective disorder, which makes her want to hibernate from October until Easter. Everything feels like an effort during those dark, wet months. "I don't take pleasure," she says, "in the things that I usually enjoy doing." She has signed up for aerobics classes in the past, but her enthusiasm sagged after a few sessions. She could walk on her own, but without a commitment spurring her onward, she would likely open the door and say, "I'm nae going out in that." The group walk ensures that Kennedy will have company and get exercise. "It makes me feel like I've done something with my day," she says, "and that gives me energy to do other things."

We reach a footpath that meanders alongside the White Cart

Water, a tributary of the Clyde. Purple-flowered buddleia hangs off the wrought-iron fence and red-brick wall that border the trail. The rain has dissipated into a light mist. My mood, too, has lifted — from the walking, sure, but mostly from the companionship.

The link between isolation and well-being should not be overlooked. The average household in the U.K. has 2.4 people, virtually the same as in the U.S. and Canada. Fifty years ago, it was 3.1 (and higher in North America). Increasingly, we rely on digital technology for community and commerce, and spend long stretches of time alone. In parts of the U.K., this is the biggest health issue faced by seniors. "Persistent loneliness leaves a mark via stress hormones, immune function and cardiovascular function," Britain's Mental Health Foundation noted in a 2010 study, "with a cumulative effect that means being lonely or not is equivalent in impact to being a smoker or non-smoker." So, it's not only sitting — *isolation* is the new smoking? Relax. Walking is an antidote here too.

Just before my trip to Scotland, Paths for All released a social return on investment (SROI) analysis of the Glasgow Health Walks program. It looked at 33 open walks (which anybody can join) and 26 closed walks aimed at hospital in-patients, people with learning disabilities, members of ethnic minorities and individuals referred by medical practitioners. In one year, nearly £50,000 was spent on staff salaries, volunteer training and other expenses. For every £1 invested, the report determined, £8 in benefits were returned to society. By making people more fit and improving their mental health, the walks helped the National Health Service and Glasgow city council reduce their spending on home care and other medical interventions, including prescriptions. In the SROI survey, more than 90 percent of walkers said they are now more confident, experience less isolation and are willing to embrace new experiences. Others reported a stronger connection to their neighbourhoods, and a better understanding of ethnicity and disability. "There is ample justification for supporting led Health Walks for the improvements they make to health and well-being alone," said the report. "However, when other benefits they deliver are included, such as improvements in cultural awareness and inclusion, the case becomes truly compelling."

Walk for half an hour, five times a week, says an American educational alliance called Every Body Walk!, and the endorphin boost will ease stress, anger and confusion. Going on a stroll "with good company and in pleasant surroundings" can ward off depression and anxiety, counsels the Canadian Centre for Occupational Health and Safety.

Probing deeper, scientists believe that walking could help forestall brain shrinkage and, in turn, dementia and Alzheimer's disease. Better circulation in the body sends more oxygen, glucose and other vital substances to the brain. In a large study of men and women in their 70s, Alan Gow, a psychology professor at Heriot-Watt University in Edinburgh, used magnetic resonance imaging (MRI) to show that septuagenarians who walked regularly experienced less white-matter atrophy. White matter is a tissue that contains nerve fibres and a type of fat called myelin, which influences the speed of nerve signalling. Other stimulating behaviours, such as playing complex games or visiting friends, did not preserve the tissue as well as walking.

A healthy brain can slow the progression of both mild cognitive impairment and Alzheimer's, according to a paper published by University of Pittsburgh cellular and molecular pathologist Cyrus Raji. At the midpoint of a 20-year study, 299 healthy men and women in their late 70s and early 80s and 127 seniors with some degree of cognitive dysfunction were given MRIs and a written questionnaire known as the mini–mental state exam (MMSE). In the latter group, men and women who walked at least five miles a week maintained brain volume (shrinkage indicates that cells are dying) and experienced less cognitive decline, as determined by the MMSE. Among healthy subjects, six miles each week made a difference.

An estimated 5.2 million Americans had Alzheimer's in 2013, costing the country more than $200 billion. As the population ages and more people are diagnosed with the disease, this figure is expected to rise to $1.2 trillion by 2050. It is the sixth-leading cause of death in the U.S., and the only cause in the top 10 without an effective medical treatment to slow its advance. The same demographic avalanche threatens much of the Western world. "Alzheimer's is a devastating illness, and unfortunately, walking is not a cure," says Raji. "But it can improve your brain's resistance to the disease and reduce memory loss over time." Regular exercise, such as walking, could reduce your risk of developing Alzheimer's by as much as 50 percent.

We shouldn't need another peer-reviewed article to convince us that walking is good for the brain, and that doing it in a natural environment — ideally, with friends — is even better. Academic work in this area, as one Scottish scientist told me, could be dismissed as research from the School of the Blindingly Obvious. First of all, we know that moderate exercise is almost universally good for our bodies. Second, we're genetically predisposed to be in nature, and when we walk in a green place, laboratory evidence has shown that stress levels fall. The body's stress response — a physiological reaction to a perceived threat, which includes a faster heart rate, faster breathing and a jolt of glucose from the liver for extra energy — is typically less pronounced in a natural setting. Remaining in a state of high alert, as one might be if on a busy street or in a bustling office all day, takes its toll. Nature can help us unwind and recharge. Still, there are dozens of ongoing investigations that could further elucidate the relationship between walking and mental health, and add precision to our understanding. So the day after my outing with Macleod's group, I am covered in rain gear and hurrying through a downpour to the University of Glasgow's main campus to meet a man who has promised to explain why this matters.

Rich Mitchell, tall and thin, with close-cropped hair and a soft English accent, is an epidemiologist at the university's Institute for Health and Wellbeing, and co-director of the Centre for Research on Environment, Society and Health, which explores how physical and social environments can influence population health, for better and for worse. He is also a Paths for All board member. I contacted Mitchell after reading a paper of his on the impact of physical activity in a natural environment. The study used data from the same Scottish Health Survey that painted a picture of the Glasgow effect. It concluded that regular exercise in a park or forest may halve your risk of suffering from poor mental health. If they make these activities a habit, people with ailments such as mild depression are better able to cope with what Mitchell calls "struggles in general life." Working out in a gym or on city streets does not have the same impact. "I wasn't surprised by the findings," he said when the study was published, "but I was surprised by just how much better it is for your mental health to exercise in a green place."

Mitchell wanted to take me for a hike in the windswept heights west of Glasgow, which look down upon the Clyde as it widens and flows toward the sea. I saw these hills yesterday from the rise in the middle of Queen's Park, but today they're blanketed by thick cloud, and judging from the torrents of rainwater flowing in the gutter beside the road, the trails would be slick with mud. Instead, he opens an oversized green-and-white umbrella and leads me through the gates of the Botanic Gardens.

Born and raised in southwestern England, near Dartmoor National Park, Mitchell spent as much time as he could walking in the hills while growing up. He began his career looking into regional health inequalities. As associate director of the Research Unit in Health and Behavioural Change at the University of Edinburgh's medical school, he spent a lot of time monitoring and measuring health indicators, and then agitating (his word) for change. "We understood that the primary drivers of these health gaps," he says, "are the social and economic difference between people's lives." As stated in the World Health Organization's 2003 report on the social determinants of health (a.k.a. *The Solid Facts*), "While medical care can prolong survival and improve prognosis after some serious diseases, more important for the health of the population as a whole are the social and economic conditions that make people ill and in need of medical care in the first place."

Mitchell agitated for several years, then began to get depressed.

He and his colleagues were deconstructing problems and suggesting solutions. But these recommendations, he says, "were really about a pretty radical reorganization of society and economy. Whilst I still think those things are what you need to do if you want to narrow health inequalities, the reality is, that's very unlikely to happen, at least in a planned way. People are unlikely to vote for some massive social and economic revolution."

If aliens landed on earth, Mitchell believes, they would quickly realize that what humanity needs is a soft transition to a "nicer" world. Yet that idea, he knows, underestimates the ability of powerful people to maintain the structures that feed their egos and wealth, and the ability of innovation and new technologies (such as fracking for natural gas) to nourish fundamentally unsustainable lifestyles. "Eventually," he says, "we won't be able to kick the ball any farther." On the other hand, he adds with a grin, "maybe next week there will be a global pandemic!" Geomorphology, the study of landforms and the processes that shape them, the foundation of his training as a geographer, teaches us that most things — for instance, a river basin — change very slowly, although events like massive floods can alter our planet very quickly.

Around the time that he was coming to these realizations, Mitchell was invited by the U.K. Forestry Commission to participate in a gathering of researchers under the auspices of a pan-European intergovernmental organization called Cooperation in Science and Technology, which aims to reduce the fragmentation of nationally funded research projects by supporting a wider, continental perspective. The objective of the project that he joined was to learn more about what forests, trees and natural places could do for the well-being of Europeans. Something clicked. Looking to test his ideas in a place that had experienced a significant amount of economic decline for a long time, he relocated to Glasgow.

Research into the curative properties of nature has been gaining momentum over the past three decades. As we splash along the tree-lined walkways of the Botanic Gardens, past a 200-year-old weeping ash, thick green hedges and roses from around the world, Mitchell gives me a crash course on environmental psychology, starting with a landmark paper published in *Science* in 1984. "View Through a Window May Influence Recovery from Surgery," by American health care–design researcher Roger Ulrich, demonstrated that patients convalescing from the surgical removal of their gallbladders had less complications, shorter post-operative hospital stays, fewer negative evaluative comments from nurses and took fewer doses of analgesics if their rooms looked out onto a natural view as opposed to a brick wall.

Five years later, in their book *The Experience of Nature: A Psychological Perspective*, University of Michigan psychology professors Rachel and Stephen Kaplan outlined their influential Attention Restoration Theory, which holds that people are able to concentrate better after they spend time in a natural setting or simply look at images of natural scenes. The Kaplans did pioneering research on soft fascination, a state in which the natural environment — clouds, rivers, leaves blowing in a breeze — holds your interest in an undramatic fashion. Because you are paying involuntary or effortless attention, not consciously focusing on something, it's possible to simultaneously reflect on your surroundings and explore other thoughts. Moreover, the serenity you derive from nature can take the sting out of any confusing or troubling "cognitive residue" your mind is churning through, an "internal noise" that can muddle acuity. "All fascinations are not equally effective," the Kaplans write. "Nature settings and activities that involve the natural environment lend themselves to restoration. Though experiences may differ in scale, they have some properties in common . . . they concern both the physical and the mental world at the same time." Basically, *being* somewhere while *doing* something produces a multiplier effect, the Kaplans argue, because humans are conceptual thinkers, and are "very good at imagining themselves going places and doing things." This is why going for a walk in the park at lunch can help you remedy a conflict back at the office.

In 2003, another American psychologist, Terry Hartig, applied this theory directly to walking. More than 100 young adults walked along a well-graded dirt road through the oak-sycamore woodland at the base of a canyon in a wilderness reserve southeast of Los Angeles. Another cohort walked through a medium-density office and retail development in the nearby city of Orange, a landscape of restaurants and shopping malls, and streets that carry an average of 24,000 vehicles each day. In addition to monitoring ambulatory blood pressure before, during and after these walks — a method that records levels at regular intervals to avoid the "white coat effect" that makes people nervous and inflates results when that cuff is pumped tight around your arm in a clinical setting — researchers had study subjects complete attentionally demanding tasks. In one, they were asked to quickly search for five target letters in a line of letters, with accuracy and speed a measure of their performance. This was a conservative assessment of Attention Restoration Theory, Hartig notes. Extreme examples of natural beauty and urban blight were not selected as the field sites. Yet the results were unequivocal. Walking in the wilderness reserve lowered blood pressure (i.e., stress) more than it did in the city, and scores on the attentional tests improved on the nature walks while declining in the urban setting. "For urban populations in particular, easy pedestrian and visual access to natural settings can produce preventive benefits," he concludes. "Public health strategies with a natural environment component may have particular value in this time of growing urban populations, exploding health care expenditures, and deteriorating environmental quality."

This statement meshes well with a British literature review published in 2012. Physical activity has been shown to alleviate the symptoms of people with mild depression, the paper noted, but its authors wanted to find out whether "the less vigorous activity of walking — a potentially widely acceptable and safe intervention — confers such benefit." After sifting through nearly 15,000 studies in 11 research databases, they determined that "walking has a statistically significant, large effect on the symptoms of depression in some populations, but the current evidence . . . is limited. Thus, while walking is a promising treatment for depression . . . with few, if any, contraindications, further investigations to establish the frequency, intensity, duration and type(s) of effective walking interventions, particularly in primary care populations, would be beneficial for providing further recommendations to clinical practitioners."

Mitchell is advancing this research front. Green space can reduce stress in deprived communities, he documented in a 2011 experiment that relied on salivary cortisol measurements, which are easily obtained by asking subjects to spit into a test tube. The body's stress response is driven by the adrenal glands. By looking at levels of cortisol, the main hormone produced by the glands, scientists can get an accurate chemical picture of how people are feeling. This was an exploratory study, with a limited sample size, and the results were modest. But, as Mitchell points out, making a small impact on a large number of people can be very important.

Picking up where that paper left off, he has launched a major project seeking empirical evidence on how walking can help people cope with the friction of daily life. Conducted with colleagues from throughout the U.K., the £950,000 study will assess the psychological impacts of Forestry Commission Scotland's Woods In and Around Towns (WIAT) improvement program. It is an attempt to determine whether contact with nature has stronger impacts on people who are confronting financial, domestic and other difficulties. Healthy and fit middle-class people might really enjoy time in nature, says Mitchell, but they won't necessarily get massive tangible benefits from a walk in the woods, just as athletes won't get into better shape from a half-hour daily stroll. On the other hand, an activity like this could have a profound effect on someone who is poor and unhappy. "That's of real interest to me," he says. "It's so hard to tackle the problems that these sorts of people face. We've tried loads of different things, and nothing has worked really well."

The WIAT project is tapping into a Forestry Commission program to improve the urban woodlands in communities that are in the bottom third of Scotland's socio-economic rankings. The chosen areas, says Mitchell, are "scrubby, nasty, hard to get into, threatening, maybe a bit dangerous." Paths and signage and other landscaping will make them more welcoming. There are three intervention sites and three comparison sites, matched according to woodland and demographic characteristics; all are neighbourhoods in cities with long histories of economic decline, and all are located in Scotland's central belt, which runs between Glasgow and Edinburgh. (Their locations are secret, for now.) After the improvements, promotional programs will be launched in the neighbourhoods around the intervention sites. Guided walks and other activities for families and children will be organized, and leaflets and other materials will be distributed, encouraging people to venture onto the trails. The control sites will be left alone, although they could receive funding for improvements at a later date. The stress levels of more than 2,000 people who live within one mile of the six woodlands will be measured. Subjects were surveyed in 2013, before the improvements were started; a year later, after the work was done; and will be surveyed again in 2015, following the social intervention phase. Data analysis is under way and results are still pending, but in the meantime, Mitchell has published a pair of papers concluding that people who made long visits to urban green space had lower rates of depression, and that adolescents exposed to urban green space exhibited less aggressive behaviour.

"What we're looking for is a change in the levels of stress in these communities," says Mitchell, as well as whether people actually use the woodlands, and whether their general orientation to nature has changed. "It will be really interesting to see what the results are. Because on the one hand, you have reasonably strong evidence from non-real-world studies about what sorts of changes will occur. But these are communities that are facing a lot of difficulties. What should we expect?

"We're asking quite a lot of nature," he adds. "We need to be careful not to overestimate what it can achieve. Nature is not a magic bullet. But for some people, it can be quite transformative."

United States Air Force medic Sharon Smith flew into Iraq on a C-130 turboprop with the 1st Marine Division during Operation Desert Storm. Twenty-three at the time, she patched up American combat casualties and injured Iraqi prisoners on the front lines. More than 20 years later, she tears up when talking about what she saw. "Sometimes it's just really difficult," she says, her voice breaking. "You come back . . . damaged." So she decided to take a very long walk.

In the spring of 2013, Smith and 13 other American war veterans set out to thru-hike the Appalachian Trail, a 2,180-mile-long footpath stretching from Springer Mountain, Georgia, to Katahdin, Maine. They were supported by a program started by Sean Gobin, an ex-Marine who had completed the trail the previous year. After two tours of Iraq and a year in Afghanistan, Gobin had four and a half months to kill between retirement from the military and the start of grad school. A tank officer on the 350-mile-long firefight from the Kuwait border to Baghdad in March 2003 — "made it to the capital," he recalls matter-of-factly, "toppled the regime" — he also played Russian roulette with IED-planting insurgents in Fallujah for seven months. Although he did not see a psychiatrist or psychologist, Gobin was concerned about the "death spiral" he had watched fellow vets fall into upon returning home.

Soldiers go back and forth between domestic normalcy and the ugliness of war, then become civilians for good and sometimes lose their ability to activate the mental switch that helped them focus on the job during each deployment. Traumatic memories play in a loop. Cynicism festers. Vets pull away from family and friends. They obsessively recheck doors and windows whenever they hear a strange sound at home, and sit with their backs to the wall at restaurants. There are flashbacks and angry outbursts. Emotional numbness. Guilt. The anguish, regardless of whether it's diagnosed as post-traumatic stress disorder, becomes internalized. Some self-medicate with alcohol or drugs. The problems get worse.

Since 2001, more than 2.5 million American men and women have returned from wars in Iraq and Afghanistan, and around 20 percent suffer from PTSD. Although smaller in scale, the stats are similar in the U.K. and Canada, where four veterans of the conflict in Afghanistan committed suicide in a single week in late 2013. PTSD, which was added to the American Psychiatric Association's *Diagnostic and Statistical Manual of Mental Disorders* in 1980, can affect anyone who experiences trauma: victims of rape, child abuse, car accidents, natural disasters. "The risk of exposure to trauma has been a part of the human condition since we evolved as a species," says the U.S. Department of Veterans Affairs. "Attacks by saber tooth tigers or 21st-century terrorists have probably produced similar psychological sequelae in the survivors of such violence."

But soldiers are particularly susceptible. "War drains your faith in humanity," says Gobin. "You come home, disassociate and disconnect, and live in a world of grey."

As a kid, he had cruised up and down the east coast in an RV with his parents, camping in national parks on the shoulders on the Appalachian Trail. He read Bill Bryson's *A Walk in the Woods*, a definitive account of the monotony, challenge and ecstasy of hiking under a heavy load day after day after day. "Distance changes utterly when you take the world on foot. . . . The world, you realize, is enormous in a way that only you and a small community of fellow hikers know," writes Bryson. "Life takes on a neat simplicity, too. Time ceases to have any meaning. When it is dark, you go to bed, and when it is light again you get up, and everything in between is just in between. It's quite wonderful, really. You have no engagements, commitments, obligations, or duties; no special ambitions and only the smallest, least complicated of wants; you exist in a tranquil tedium, serenely beyond the reach of exasperation, 'far removed from the seats of strife,' as the early explorer and botanist William Bartram put it. All that is required of you is a willingness to trudge."

Gobin was ready to trudge. Fellow ex-Marine Mark Silvers, his trail-mate, wanted to hike the Appalachian Trail as a fundraiser, so the pair planned informal gatherings at Veterans of Foreign Wars (VFW) posts in towns along the route to collect donations for disabled soldiers. At some stops, 200 people showed up. At others, they spent the evening throwing back cheap whisky and trading war stories with a couple of old-timers. Descending Mount Katahdin, they had pledges totalling $50,000, which were put toward the purchase of three handicap-accessible vehicles for seriously wounded veterans.

Gobin and Silvers were overwhelmed by the reception they received in trail towns. Locals offered meals and drives to help them run errands. Vietnam vets shook their hands and said, "I know what you're going through. There's a light at the end of the tunnel." On the trail, they hung out with other thru-hikers, most of whom were vastly different than the type of people one encounters in the military, an important part of the socialization process for soldiers with PTSD, who might otherwise avoid contact with strangers. Physically, they got into great shape. Daily 15-mile hikes are more gruelling than anything you do in the military, says Gobin, and a lot of people let themselves go after discharge, gaining weight and losing self-esteem.

"A long-distance hike reveals character," he says. "People have bad days. You're dealing with your own struggles, the weather, the terrain. How you cope with that and interact with other people facilitates personal development. If you're in a group, you try to help others when they're down. That helps you regain a sense of camaraderie, that feeling of being on a mission, which gives you a sense of purpose again."

Mostly, though, hiking all day every day, week after week, you attain soft fascination. You relive your combat experiences 100 times each day while in this soothing state, and you have time to process the memories. "Out in nature for so long," says Gobin, "you have a chance to think about what's important, about what you want to do next. Toward the end of the trail, I realized how beautiful the country is. The colour came back to my life."

The Appalachian Trail Conservancy, the not-for-profit that manages and maintains the footpath, was watching his fundraiser. The organization was looking for a way to honour the memory of Earl Shaffer, a World War II vet who, in 1948, became the first person to thru-hike the route that officially became the A.T. when President Lyndon B. Johnson signed into law the National Trails System Act in 1968. Shaffer had served in the U.S. Army Signal Corps in the South Pacific. He told a friend he wanted to "walk off" the sights and sounds of battle, and did the trail in five months, without a guidebook or any of the lightweight gear that walkers depend on today. The A.T. Conservancy contacted Gobin, and his Warrior Hike program was born. Its aim is simple: help veterans struggling with PTSD turn a corner on their trauma.

Gobin built a website and a schedule for the 2013 thru-hike, organizing stops at VFW posts as he and Silvers had done. Within two weeks, 13 vets applied, men and women ranging in age from 26 to 50. Like Sharon Smith, all met the program's criteria: they needed help. Gobin called every outdoor company and retailer he could think of, asking them to donate tents, backpacks and other gear. The supplies were sent directly to Springer Mountain, and he drove down from the University of Virginia, in Charlottesville, hiking with the group for the first two weeks before returning to campus for year-end exams in his MBA program.

The weather that spring was terrible. Storms blanketed the trail with snow in the mountain ranges of North Carolina. Then it rained for weeks. Norovirus swept through the group. One hiker got kidney stones. Another needed an emergency appendectomy. When they reached New York, a heat wave hit. The humidity was crushing. Some veterans made poor decisions, and very quickly learned from them. They were drinking and partying and falling behind. And then they asked: What am I getting out of this? Maybe drinking isn't important. Maybe doing something bigger than myself is more important.

"It was pandemonium," says Gobin, who coordinated the walk from his home, stuck on the couch with his laptop. In the end, only Smith and five others completed the hike. The reasons people dropped out varied, from injuries to spouses needing them back. Still, when asked in a follow-up survey how the experience improved their mental well-being, on a scale of one to 10, with 10 being "immensely,"

Warrior Hikers reported an average score of 9.5. Smith cherished the opportunity to spend time alone with her thoughts and the support she received from the people she met along the way.

The program expanded in 2014. In addition to the A.T., Gobin sent groups onto the Pacific Crest Trail and Continental Divide Trail, which together comprise the Triple Crown of American long-distance hikes. He also partnered with Georgia Southern University psychologist Shauna Joye and PhD candidate Zachary Dietrich. Both ex-military themselves, Joye and Dietrich spent a couple days on the A.T. with walkers and, afterwards, provided tele-therapy counselling. Their goal was to help vets recognize PTSD triggers and learn coping techniques.

All that time walking slowly with no distractions, says Dietrich, allows people to get deep into their own headspace, to diagnose problems and, with proper guidance, to devise solutions. An avid hiker, accustomed to solitude on his home trail, the Knobstone, in southern Indiana, Dietrich knows the power of the "green blur" that settles in after a few hours alone in the forest. Research has found that thinking about a traumatic event can be therapeutic, adds Joye, although this can be a bit of a tightrope: too much rumination can be detrimental to recovery. Hence their decision to provide counselling to Warrior Hikers, to lean on the formulaic nature of cognitive behavioural therapy (i.e., there's not much talk of dreams) to help men and women forget about the stigma around "shrinks" and the military's doctrine of macho stoicism. Ultimately, they will publish a paper examining the benefits of long-distance hiking for veterans with PTSD. And though it's not practical to think that thousands of vets will spend six months walking, there are hundreds of 40-, 50- and 60-mile-long trails throughout the United States. The possibilities for shorter excursions are endless.

Seriously injured soldiers cannot hike, so Gobin is looking at adding a cross-country bicycle trip and maybe a paddling expedition down the Mississippi. He has also been talking to a DEA agent — first-responders, including firefighters, experience a lot of PTSD

— and someone who runs a shelter for women who have been victims of violence. "There's a whole other segment of society that could benefit from this," he says. "It's bigger than just veterans."

Depression and anxiety are often dismissed as luxury disorders, as First World problems. If you are worried about when you will next eat, or where you will sleep, or who might attack in the night, your brain is probably too busy for existential dread. This is not entirely true. Although rates of mental illness in the U.S. are among the highest on the planet, in 2012 the World Health Organization reported that more than 350 million people globally suffer from depression, the leading cause of disability worldwide. Relative disparity is one of the causes, according to Ron Kessler, the Harvard Medical School professor who led the WHO's research. If your house is worth $400,000, but all of your neighbours live in million-dollar mansions, you may feel inadequate. If you have one goat and your neighbours have a flock, same thing. But there are other factors — like our sedentary lives. "Preventing depression increasingly appears to be a question of movement," Sarah Goodyear writes on the *Atlantic*'s CityLab website, "the kind of movement that humans evolved to perform and that is eliminated from everyday life by machines, hired labor, and automobiles."

Inactive mice are more anxious than mice with exercise wheels in their cages, according to a Princeton University study. The runners demonstrated a greater willingness to explore — a sign of confidence — and their brains produced more of a neurotransmitter called GABA, which helps the animals remain calm. When dunked in ice-cold water for five minutes, a bath that mice do not enjoy, the active mice recovered more quickly from the stress than the sedentary control group. These results corroborate studies that show how exercise reduces anxiety in humans, says Princeton psychologist Elizabeth Gould. For instance, a Swedish experiment which determined that people engaging in two hours of light physical activity (walking, gardening) each week had a 63 percent reduced risk of developing depression. And they support the declarations of experts such as John Arden, the director of mental-health training at American health-care provider Kaiser Permanente: "Walking is the cheapest and easiest way to get relief from depression."

Mark Norwine knows this territory better than most. In April 2013, after a series of suicides at Missouri high schools, the 54-year-old bullying-prevention coordinator at a non-profit mental-health coalition embarked on a 200-mile walk across the state on the Katy Trail, one of American's longest rails-to-trails conversion projects. Norwine, who had been diagnosed with bipolar disorder two years earlier, stopped to talk at schools in small towns along the route — communities that lack the resources to address mental-health concerns among teenagers. Even if they had the capacity, there is still a taboo to overcome.

When he was growing up, nobody talked about cancer, Norwine says in one packed school gym, a scene captured in the documentary film about his journey, *Walking Man*. Then AIDS received the silent treatment. Today, even though unchecked mental illness heightens the risk of alcohol and drug abuse, divorce, poverty, prison and homelessness, we tend to not talk about it openly. "'Tough it out,'" says Joseph Parks, the chief clinical director of the Missouri Department of Mental Health, summarizing the prevailing attitude in rural areas. "'We're individualistic out here. Every man for himself.' That ideology is good for business, but not for somebody who is depressed and thinking about killing himself."

Throughout his life, Norwine surfed the peaks and troughs of depression. He lost his job frequently and had trouble finishing anything. After a string of sleepless nights, delivering newspapers on a dark highway, he almost died in a car crash. Working with troubled teens became part of his therapy. At each stop on the walk, he broke the taboo. He told students what symptoms to watch for and where they could seek help. Like Stanley Vollant's audience, the kids listened.

Norwine's son Eric, who has also been diagnosed with bipolar disorder, joined Mark on the trek. The condition is hereditary — a couple of cousins shot themselves. It will likely always be part of the Norwines' lives. But physical activity keeps it at bay. Mark's sneakers are as important as his pills. Going for a walk every morning on the streets around his suburban St. Louis home gives him strength to face the rest of the day, to get through the dark winter. And in the spring, on the green ribbon of the Katy Trail, travelling with his son, and a purpose, Mark felt the stirrings of Rebecca Solnit's three-note chord. After 17 days, for one of the first times in his life, he finished what he started.

"I don't know what my future holds," Eric, now in his mid-20s, says at the end of the documentary. "But what walking with my dad has taught me is that if I grow up to be anything like him, I think I'll be okay."

Duke University neuroscientist James Blumenthal was one of the first to study the impact of exercise on depression. His groundbreaking research in the late 1990s demonstrated that activities such as brisk walking relieved the symptoms of major depression just as effectively as drug therapy, and that sustained exercise prevented the pain from returning.

In one experiment, 156 patients were divided into three groups. Men and women in the first were treated with the antidepressant drug sertraline, better known by its trade name Zoloft (more than 37 million Zoloft prescriptions were written in the U.S. in 2011 — 13 million more than Prozac, but 10 million fewer than the anti-anxiety drug Xanax). Patients in the second group took the same dosage of sertraline and exercised three times a week for 45 minutes: 10 minutes of warm-up, half an hour of walking or light jogging, a five-minute cool-down. Group three just exercised. After 16 weeks of supervised treatment, patients in all three cohorts showed similar improvement. Eighty-three, distributed evenly across the groups, were declared free from depression. But when Blumenthal checked in with those patients six months later, with no additional treatment in the interim, 38 percent of people in the medication-only group had relapsed, as had 31 percent in the medication and exercise group, while only 8 percent in the exercise-only group had slipped back into depression. "One of the positive psychological benefits of systematic exercise," Blumenthal and his co-authors wrote in a paper about the experiment, "is the development of a sense of personal mastery and positive self-regard."

Walking can do more than boost confidence. It has been shown to promote new links between different parts of the brain, and to stimulate the growth of neurons and their ability to transmit messages. This can improve our memories and our ability to focus on complex ideas — it helps our brains navigate the intellectual puzzles of daily life.

Seven hundred miles northwest of Duke, at the University of Illinois in Urbana-Champaign, Chuck Hillman's Neurocognitive Kinesiology Laboratory uses electroencephalography (EEG) and functional MRI (fMRI) to look at brain activity during exercise. The brain's cells communicate through electrical impulses; electrodes attached to the scalp can capture an EEG recording. Blood flows into parts of the brain that are in use, and fMRI measures neural activity by detecting changes in blood flow. Hillman, whose PhD is in clinical psychology, is most interested in childhood health. One of his studies, published in 2005, was the first to use neural-imaging tools to investigate connections between fitness and cognitive behaviour among kids. Verbal and math test results, as well as other performance measures, all improved with exercise. Treadmills and stationary bicycles in classrooms have been shown to help children concentrate and learn. He wanted to know why.

The 2005 study found that aerobic fitness was linked to behavioural performance in preadolescent children. In the decade since then, Hillman's work has confirmed that there is a causal relationship between brain activation and walking. In one experiment, children walked moderately for 20 minutes without breaking a sweat. EEG images showed a burst of activity in the prefrontal cortex while they walked, and the neurons continued firing for at least an hour after they stopped moving. The prefrontal cortex manages a function called executive control. Essentially, it governs our ability to remain focused, our working memory and our cognitive flexibility. Executive control helps students pay attention, retain and manipulate information, and multitask. The prefrontal cortex lights up when we walk, and we are better able to perform complex tasks. Hillman, who has authored nearly 100 papers, has shown that even a single 20-minute bout of exercise can improve the scholastic performance of students with attention deficit hyperactivity disorder (ADHD).

In the United States, the No Child Left Behind policy, an act of Congress that ties school funding to the achievement of basic academic skills, has led 44 percent of administrators to cut gym and recess time in favour of more reading and mathematics. As a result, in 2011, nearly 60 percent of students did not attend a physical education class in an average week. "That's completely the wrong message," says Hillman. "We need to be adding *more* physical activity. Not only because we have an obesity epidemic, but also because it's very clear there are benefits to cognitive function, memory and learning." By serving on committees with organizations such as the National Academy of Sciences, he strives to get his data and similar findings into the hands of policy-makers, "to enhance their understanding that physical activity is important not just for physical health but also mental health.

"People always say to me, 'That's obvious. Exercise is good for the brain.' But how obvious is it? And if it's so obvious, how come there's no concern for people's brain health, outside of concussions? You don't hear, 'I'm concerned about your brain, so let's go get some exercise.'"

In the U.S., 11 percent of children between the ages of four and 17 were diagnosed with ADHD in 2011, up from 9.5 percent in 2007 and 7.8 percent in 2003, according to the Centers for Disease Control and Prevention. ADHD is the second most common long-term diagnosis among children, trailing only asthma. More than half of these children — about 3.5 million — are on medication. Pharmaceutical companies earned nearly $9 billion from the sale of stimulant drugs to Americans in 2012. They fund comic books that market the meds directly to kids. "Medicines may make it easier to pay attention and control your behavior!" says a superhero subsidized by the multinational Shire. One of its main products is Adderall, marketed not only as a way to control ADHD but also to boost academic performances, a claim backed by studies funded by Shire. And now adult ADHD is a growing market for drug companies; almost 16 million prescriptions were written for Americans in their 20s and 30s in 2012, a dramatic rise from 5.6 million in 2007. Psychologist Keith Connors, a pioneering ADHD researcher and an early advocate for the recognition and pharmaceutical treatment of the condition, has done an about-face. "The numbers make it look like an epidemic. Well, it's not. It's preposterous," the professor emeritus at Duke told the *New York Times*. "This is a concoction to justify the giving out of medication at unprecedented and unjustifiable levels."

In 2013, a British company called Intelligent Health, which works with public and private partners to counter inactivity, conducted an experiment in which 2,500 seven- and eight-year-olds began walking to school. Eighty percent of the children reported that they felt calmer and were better able to focus on their lessons. Family doctor William Bird, the company's director, believes that something this simple could help wean us off Ritalin and other drugs used to treat ADHD, which cost England's National Health Service more than £30 million in prescriptions every year. "Chronic stress leads to inactivity and creates more chronic stress," he wrote in the *Economist*. "Chronic stress leads to the desire to consume high calorie foods since the body thinks it is preparing for a bad time ahead. Chronic stress increases the need for immediate gratification of smoking, alcohol and drugs as a way to cope with this never-ending anxiety and low grade fear."

In his book *Mad Travelers: Reflections on the Reality of Transient Mental Illnesses*, Canadian philosopher Ian Hacking explores a brief epidemic of hysterical fugue, or compulsive wandering, that broke out in Europe in the late 1800s. Albert Dadas, a part-time gas company worker in Bordeaux, France, "deserted family, work, and daily life to walk as fast as he could, straight ahead, sometimes doing 70 kilometres a day on foot," according to the notes of his physician. "In the end he would be arrested for vagrancy and thrown in prison." (The condition is also known as dromomania — from the Greek words for *running* and *insanity* — or, in French, *automatisme ambulatoire*.)

Dadas walked obsessively, without any apparent motivation or destination. Reports of his journeys set off a small wave that spread to Italy, Germany and Russia. Hacking labels hysterical fugue a "transient mental illness," its incidence restricted to a specific place and time, in this case less than 25 years. *Mad Travelers* argues that some ailments, including ADHD and chronic fatigue, could be the products of an "ecological niche" — and that we may be laying the temporal groundwork for other "mental illnesses of the moment."

My obsession, in this light, can be seen as more than a Luddite's flight from mid-life ennui. It could have been spurred by the conflux of rabid consumerism and technological utopianism. By the acceleration of the Anthropocene. Discord at work and a torn meniscus were only the final straws. And I am not alone.

The helpful spiders of Google Alert, which scour English-language news sites around the world and send me a daily email with dozens of links to stories related to walking, invariably uncover people on long treks, on every continent except Antarctica. (Most of the headlines, mind you, are about the television series *The Walking Dead*, and about pedestrians hit and killed by vehicles while walking beside American highways.) Many dromomaniacs walk to raise awareness about a particular disease, or to raise funds for a worthy cause. Others walk to lose weight. To remember a deceased child. To forget a bad marriage. For adventure. For some, it's a spiritual pilgrimage — another subject for a later chapter. But I suspect there might be a little bit of pathological wanderlust behind each journey.

Nearly 30 percent of Europe's adult population experiences at least one mental-health problem every year, it is estimated, and the annual cost of poor mental health in Scotland is £10.7 billion. Epidemiologist Rich Mitchell calls this *the* biggest public health challenge on the continent. "That's why the potential for contact with nature is so important," he says. "It's very hard to think about how you can tackle that level of population health problem from solely a service base, such as doctors prescribing things, or people being treated in some sort of formal, clinical way. I don't think that type of approach would be.sustainable."

Although Mitchell believes the publicly funded care provided by Britain's National Health Service is "brilliant" for acute problems like heart attacks and car crashes, he feels that it stumbles when dealing with chronic health issues, particularly those associated with an aging population, especially for people who have several things wrong with them. Like Dr. Michael Evans in Toronto, he doesn't have much confidence in the ability of the pharmaceutical industry to steer us clear of these long-term problems: "My standard, cynical line is that basically what they want is for the population to be sick enough to need their medicine but not to die. Because once they die, they stop being a source of money. Some of these chronic health issues are a pharmaceutical company's dream. Clearly, there's a profit motive. That's what capitalism does."

The most basic goal of his research, on the other hand, is to introduce the idea that contact with and activity in nature could improve public health and, potentially, "narrow the health gap between rich and poor people." He wants to constantly feed this possibility into the minds of physicians, health-care planners and anybody else remotely concerned with population health. The Woods In and Around Towns project is intended to serve as a litmus test of these ideas — to find out who benefits from activity in a natural setting, who doesn't benefit and how benefits can be equalized. In the long run, he hopes his work can influence urban planning, landscape design and policy, all in the name of encouraging contact with nature and designing urban places that enable healthy living.

Mitchell has been keeping an eye on our whereabouts as we walk. My executive control has been maxed out trying to follow the arc of his research and avoid puddles while staying on pace with his long stride. No green blur for me today. After circling the Botanic Gardens, we follow a footpath alongside the rushing River Kelvin, which drains the hills north of the city. The path leads us back to the University of Glasgow campus, where he suggests we retreat to a café to dry off. One of the best things about interviewing people while walking is that you invariably end up at a pub or coffee shop.

Inside, we remove our rain gear and sit down with cappuccinos. I tell Mitchell about my mood improving after talking to others during the health walk the previous night, and he agrees that going for a "blether" with friends is one of the unsung benefits of walking. Still, the Health Walks program is a baby step toward addressing the problems in a city that he calls "the sick man of Europe." Parks and trails may help address Glasgow's woes, but another of Mitchell's goals is to challenge people "who believe that nature will save everything and everybody and all you really need to do is get people out there in the park or the woods or the mountains and everything will be all right. Because that's just not true."

He leaves me with one more caution: "Walking can be seen as egalitarian, as an activity that fosters equality. But I think you have to be careful. Inequalities do persist around who is choosing to walk, what environments are they walking in, what's the purpose of their walking. I think we need to pay attention to that. Though I've yet to see a study that says walking is detrimental for you."

three

SOCIETY

"The city is seen as serving a democratic function where people encounter social diversity and gain a greater understanding of each other by sharing the same city space."

— *Jan Gehl*, Cities for People

"If there is any way of seeing less of a country than from a motor-car, I have yet to experience it."

— *Eric Newby*, A Short Walk in the Hindu Kush

In the pre-dawn darkness of August 18, 2012, Philadelphia police officer Moses Walker, Jr., stepped out the front door of the department's 22nd District headquarters. He had just finished working an overnight shift, watching prisoners in the holding cell. Before Walker left for the bus stop, a colleague offered a ride.

"It's a nice day," he replied. "I'm going to walk."

Wearing shorts, a ball cap and a blue wind jacket, knapsack on his back, hands in his pockets, the 40-year-old headed west along Cecil B. Moore Avenue, one of the main arteries through hardscrabble North Philly. At 5:46 a.m., four blocks from the station house, two men slipped out of the shadows on the opposite side of the street.

Walker looked over his left shoulder a couple times. The pair caught up and demanded money. Instead of surrendering his wallet, the 19-year veteran, eligible for retirement in a few months, a deacon at nearby Deliverance Evangelist Church, reached for his service revolver.

He was found face down on sidewalk, bullet holes in his chest, stomach and arm, the unholstered gun beneath his body. One of three shooting deaths in Philly that night.

Nearly a year later, with the bloodstains gone and his assailants facing murder charges, I stood on the spot where Walker was attacked. It was a humid early summer afternoon. Officer Brian Nolan ducked under the branches of a young oak tree, took off his peaked blue hat and wiped the sweat from his forehead with a bare forearm. "This is a job just like any other job," he said after describing Walker's funeral, "except I could get killed."

Six feet tall and 185 pounds, with a buzz cut and a square jaw, Nolan had wanted to be a cop since he was a kid. Both of his grandfathers were police officers, and a couple of uncles too. He began his law-enforcement career in Wildwood, New Jersey, a boardwalk town on the Atlantic shore, before moving inland, across the Delaware River, to America's fifth-largest city. A minor leaguer called up to the Show. Then his professional development took a slight detour. For a full year, Nolan walked the beat in one of the most dangerous places in the country.

Until recently, as in most North American jurisdictions, new cops in Philly spent the lion's share of their patrol time driving around in cruisers. "When I started 16 years ago," one officer told me, "you came out of the academy and it was, 'Hey, rookie — here's the car keys and a map.'" Today, on the heels of a game-changing research project conducted by the city's police department and criminologists from Temple University, whose main campus is in the 22nd District, all fresh graduates begin their service on foot duty. Every shift, day or night, rain or snow, they walk.

The program — the first of its kind in the United States — appears to be successful. Preliminary statistics show that crime rates are falling. Perhaps more important, I was told, cops and citizens are starting to develop a deeper trust for one another. A trust that could help mend some of the rips in the urban fabric.

"Being human is itself difficult, and therefore all kinds of settlements (except dream cities) have problems," Jane Jacobs wrote in her most influential book, 1961's *The Death and Life of Great American Cities*. "Big cities have difficulties in abundance, because they have people in abundance." To maintain order — a marvelous, complex swirl of safety and freedom — a city must encourage "an intricacy of sidewalk use . . . a constant succession of eyes." Jacobs spoke of the way shoppers and students and seniors and police officers weave through each other's lives, completing their daily travels and tasks while sharing a ribbon of concrete, a "ballet in which the individual dancers and ensembles all have distinctive parts which miraculously reinforce each other and compose an orderly whole."

A flow of pedestrians, Jacobs and many others have argued, can help unify a city or town. When you are in a car, or online, the anonymity can breed anti-social or amoral behaviour. Road rage, mean-spirited comment threads and spur-of-the-moment crimes spill out of the same bucket. On foot, you are immersed in a multi-sensory, interactive environment, not sequestered behind one-way glass. You see and are seen, hear and are heard. Sure, you can put on blinders — headphones and smartphones drown out local frequencies — but pedestrians have more opportunities to engage and empathize with the people they pass by and live among. It could be something as fleeting as a salutatory nod or smile. Maybe a short conversation with a stranger, or a long talk with an old pal. Petting a dog. Peeking inside a store window. Reading a handmade sign on a lamppost or smelling the flowers in a front garden. Even if nobody is around, you feel an implied presence.

At home, I am razzed by retired neighbours, an ex-cop and an ex-taxman, when I walk errands in the middle of the afternoon. "How's the writing coming? So, this is considered 'research,' eh?" In North Philly, cops and robbers lob similar taunts.

"What happened?" a fleshy young man said to Nolan and his partner, Mike Farrell, as they walked past. "Somebody steal your car?"

"Just getting some exercise," Nolan shot back. "You might want to try it sometime."

The way you travel around a city impacts your impressions of other people, psychologists at the University of Surrey, in England, demonstrated in a 2012 experiment. Participants were shown an ambiguous video of two teenaged boys behaving aggressively and a teen girl texting at a nearby park bench. The video was shot four different ways: from the perspective of a driver, a transit passenger, a cyclist and a pedestrian. Study subjects who watched the driving video attributed more negative characteristics to the actors (threatening, unpleasant) than those who watched the cyclist and pedestrian videos. When observing the teens more intimately, at a slower pace, positive characteristics such as "considerate" and "well-educated" were much more likely to come to mind. People make quick judgments about their surroundings when travelling through a new environment. Drivers form a more superficial impression than pedestrians because they are exposed to less information, and because this information is gleaned in "thin slices." Our systems for interpreting sensory observations evolved to work effectively when walking. We can see other people clearly from around 300 feet away, but it takes about a minute to reach them, giving us time to assess and react to the situation.

Somebody driving along a city street past a group of teens in a park might see "a few lads who are up to no good," the study concludes. A passenger looks out the window of a bus and wonders what those young toughs are doing. A cyclist hears the boys playfully making fun of each other. A pedestrian recognizes her neighbour's son and says hello.

These casual, up-close encounters don't happen as often as they did even a generation ago, because in today's urban ecological niche, we spend so much time sitting in cars or staring at screens, or staring at screens while sitting in cars. Because we're generally in a rush.

Because we consider busyness a kind of "existential reassurance," Tim Kreider writes in the *New York Times*, "a hedge against emptiness." Because fear sells, so news broadcasts warn us to be leery of the unknown. But just as walking could help alleviate many of our mental illnesses of the moment, maybe it's also a step toward more social cohesion. Philadelphia's foot-patrol program won't bring back Moses Walker, Jr., but maybe it can help the 22nd District find a new rhythm.

Families spill off the stoops of 14-foot-wide, two-storey, red-brick row houses. Outdoor speakers blast hip hop and old-school soul. Girls wearing sundresses and flip-flops, their hair tied into braids, play with skipping ropes and dolls; boys with basketballs and toy cars. Women and men flip burgers and chicken breasts on charcoal grills. Most of their homes are small, crowded and hot, so people socialize on the streets. Wooden barricades with peeling paint stop traffic at some intersections. It's a little after noon on Saturday, and the block parties — a summer weekend ritual in North Philly — have begun.

"Yo, we got Philadelphia's finest out here today," a woman calls through an open screen door as officers Nolan and Farrell pass. "Happy Father's Day, gentlemen."

The holiday doesn't begin for nearly 12 hours, yet "Happy Father's Day" is the customary greeting. It's what you say to any man you meet.

Nolan, 24, and Farrell, 27, a firefighter for seven years before joining the force, are white. Virtually everybody else in the area is black. With guns and batons clipped to their belts, and radios emitting bursts of chatter from their shoulders, the officers walk by barbershops, corner grocers, storefront churches, parks adorned with folk-art sculptures, domino tournaments under tarp gazebos and makeshift backboards nailed to telephone poles. They kick soccer balls with kids and banter about the weather with grandmothers cradling babies on rickety front porches, ignoring the hard looks from young men with pointy beards and neck tattoos.

"Are you okay, ma'am?" Farrell asks a middle-aged woman they rouse from sleep on the steps of a shuttered shop. She is wearing a red golf shirt and has a security badge from the U.S. Open Championships on a lanyard around her neck. A city ordinance prohibits people from loitering on the property of closed businesses. "Have you been drinking? Are you diabetic? On drugs?"

"I wish I was," the woman mutters before wriggling into her shoes and staggering away.

The sun-baked sidewalks of the 22nd District are littered with broken glass, plastic baggies, cigarette butts and tufts of tobacco that have been dumped out of cigars to make nests for marijuana. Disposable cups and chip bags skitter along the pavement in the breeze. Like a mouth in desperate need of dental work, the street-scape is pocked with burned-down and boarded-up buildings, and derelict yards full of rotting couches. Moses Walker, Jr., was one of 35 people killed in the four-square-mile district in 2012, making it the city's murder capital for the third consecutive year. My own neighbourhood is roughly the same size. It hasn't seen a homicide in almost a decade.

It's tough to know where to start when listing the litany of challenges faced by families on Nolan and Farrell's turf. Poverty, unemployment, drugs, crime, racism — a lethal mix with roots that can be traced back through the 1980s crack epidemic, the 1970s heroin epidemic, the corresponding proliferations of semi-automatic weapons and handguns, and a system of real-estate segregation that started in the early 1900s, when waves of southern blacks began migrating to northern cities to escape oppression and find work. In search of a better future, hundreds of thousands ended up stuck in the ghetto.

Capt. Roland Lee, the 22nd District's commanding officer, believes that at least three-quarters of the shootings in his territory are drug-related. Low-level dealers losing their cool over a few dollars. "You stand on the corner, you fighting, and you killing each other," one former dealer said to the *Philadelphia City Paper*. "You're working for sneakers and to smoke blunts." Of the 331 homicides committed in Philadelphia in 2012 — a per capita rate roughly four times higher than New York's — 86 percent of victims were killed with guns. Like Walker and his murderers, 83 percent of the perpetrators and 80 percent of the victims were black. The City of Brotherly Love is Philadelphia's most prominent nickname (*philos*, in Greek, means love; *adelphos* is brother), but Killadelphia is more up to date.

The city's police have struggled to stop the shootings and other violent crime, even as rates fell dramatically in most large American cities over the past two decades. Their confrontational history may be part of the problem. The department's downtown headquarters, a curvilinear 1960s concrete building called the Roundhouse, resembles a pair of handcuffs when viewed from above. It's closely associated with late police-commissioner-turned-mayor Frank Rizzo, a law-and-order cop who in 1979 was charged with committing and condoning widespread and severe acts of police brutality. Six years later, officers dropped a bomb from a helicopter onto a fortified row house where members of a radical black activist organization had holed up during an armed standoff. The ensuing fire killed six adults and five children, and burned down 60 adjacent homes.

Nolan and Farrell have a kinder, gentler mission. They are here to comprehend, not apprehend. If they happen upon a crime, or spot somebody with an outstanding warrant, they will take action. But mostly, their role is simply to be a presence and a deterrence. To be approachable. To serve and protect. "Police work is basically just talking to people," says Sgt. Bisarat Worede, who supervises the 22nd District's foot beats. Nine months at the academy give you a solid base. "But in neighbourhoods like this, the real education you're going to get is from dealing with people."

Worede, whose family emigrated to the U.S. from Eritrea when he was a child, likens effective policing to following a recipe. You need to use the right amount of each ingredient, otherwise the dish won't turn out right. Foot beats aren't a panacea, he knows. Cops in cruisers can get to calls faster. And the root causes of social strife persist. But when officers walk, instead of patrolling inside 4,000 pounds of metal, they're seen as fellow human beings, even if their faces are a different colour. And because they're getting to know locals at three miles an hour, not parachuting into the middle of a crime scene, rookie cops are realizing that most people are good, even in tough parts of town.

So far, the recipe seems to be working. In 2013, there were 28 homicides in the 22nd District, seven fewer than the year before. The number of shootings also dropped (165 to 136), as did aggravated assaults (825 to 739) and burglaries (868 to 713). Of course, as the *City Paper* notes, this improvement may not last: "Murder rates fluctuate, and Philly's could spike again."

Nolan and Farrell lead me inside a crack house. The walls are punched with holes and the floors are covered with scorched Brillo pads and empty glass vials. They hear a noise upstairs and draw their revolvers, but all we see on the second floor are mouse droppings and more empty vials. We walk through a party in the courtyard of the Norman Blumberg housing project, twin towers rising above a warren of low-rise units. A gang that deals drugs out of here threatened to kill a cop this summer. Kids play; their parents barbecue and drink cocktails out of red plastic cups. In the squalid stairwell of one of the towers, which we climb slowly before descending by elevator, the smell of charcoal smoke is overpowered by urine. Although alert and watchful, Nolan and Farrell try to remain upbeat. They nod and say "Happy Father's Day" to the men who make eye contact, and most return the premature salutation. Some are not happy that the boys in blue are here.

"They got attitude. They hasslin' people that ain't causing no trouble," says Nassir Brown, sitting on a curb down the street from the Blumberg courtyard. "Yeah, we got issues here. Look at them abandoned buildings. Look at them abandoned cars. We got no jobs. Why not pay people in the community to fix things? They ain't tackling the real issues. Don't nobody in the ghetto manufacture drugs."

That's not a typical response, though — at least among the people who talk to me. A few blocks away, shaking a jug of powdered fruit punch for his kids, loud gospel music swelling out the open door, Keenan Jones spots my camera and asks if I'm a film-location scout. I explain why I'm here and ask how the foot patrols have changed his neighbourhood. "Well," he says, "me and you can talk right here right now without no gunshots going off."

Sir Robert Peel, the father of modern law enforcement, gave us the beat cop. As England's home secretary, he spearheaded the drive to establish the London Metropolitan Police in 1829. Private watchmen were replaced by professional "bobbies," a nod to Peel's first name. Military-style squads already existed elsewhere in Europe and beyond, but London's force was the first created specifically to "manage the social conflict resulting from rapid urbanization and industrialization," according to American criminologist George L. Kelling.

Policing in the United States followed the English model. The first publicly funded police departments were formed in the mid-19th century in northeastern cities such as New York and Boston. Arising out of a 200-year-old system of volunteer patrols and paid constables, the Philadelphia Police Department was founded in 1854, and its evolution reflects changes that have taken place across the country.

At first, all officers walked their beats in Philly. Ninety-three horses were purchased in 1889; motorcycles and cars were added to the fleet in 1906 and 1936, respectively. Over the decades, the role of police officers in the U.S. shifted from maintaining public order to fighting crime. And as car culture began to dominate all aspects of American life — stoking a much broader rejection of walking, especially for routine activities such as shopping and travelling to school or work — cops increasingly chased bad guys from behind the wheel. "I've always had a theory that one of the greatest inventions was police cars, because it made us more mobile," police chief Frank Hooper, of Gainsville, Georgia, told the New York Times. "And one of the worst inventions was air-conditioning, because we rolled our windows up."

As early as the 1960s, with racial tension boiling over throughout the U.S., law-enforcement reformers lobbied for a return to Peel-style policing. They wanted to see more boots on the street, and an emphasis on conversations between cops and citizens. But the prevailing wisdom held that while foot patrols improved perceptions of police and made people feel safe, they didn't actually curtail crime. One officer in a car could cover more ground than a dozen men on foot, a big consideration for cash-strapped forces.

That reliance on cars was reinforced by a 1978 study in New Jersey conducted by a team that included Kelling, who is also credited with developing the "broken window theory" — the idea that minor urban disorder, such as vandalism, paves the way for major crime — and still works as a research fellow at Harvard. The Newark Foot Patrol Experiment used special state funding to convince skeptical police chiefs to temporarily get officers out of cars and onto walking beats. "Foot patrol, in their eyes, had been pretty much discredited," Kelling writes in the *Atlantic*. "It reduced the mobility of the police, who thus had difficulty responding to citizen calls for service, and it weakened headquarters' control over patrol." The Newark study did find that residents of foot-patrolled neighbourhoods felt more secure and had a more positive impression of police, and that "officers walking beats had higher morale, greater job satisfaction, and a more favorable attitude toward citizens in their neighborhoods than did officers assigned to patrol cars." But there was no impact on crime rates. Similar experiments in Boston and Asheville, North Carolina, supported this conclusion. As recently as 2004, the U.S. National Research Council dismissed foot patrols as "an unfocused community policing strategy." And because there was no bang, there would be no more bucks.

Thirty years after the Newark study, Temple University criminologist Jerry Ratcliffe, who began his career as a bobby walking through the labyrinthine housing projects of east-end London, the poorest borough in England, got a call from Philadelphia police commissioner Charles Ramsey. Not long after he was appointed to the top position in America's fourth-largest police department,

Ramsey dispatched veteran-rookie foot patrol pairs to some of the city's most violent crime hot spots. The commissioner then asked Ratcliffe, director of Temple's Center for Security and Crime Science and a research advisor to the police department, to evaluate the initiative. Ratcliffe found that the beat cops had been effective but couldn't come up with a definitive appraisal. "If you ever do this again," he said to Ramsey, "it'd be great if you could phone us beforehand so we could help you set up something that would be really robust scientifically."

That call came in early 2009. Two hundred and forty new officers were going to graduate from the academy in a few weeks, and the commissioner wanted all of them to walk the beat.

In record time, Ratcliffe designed the Philadelphia Foot Patrol Experiment like a randomized clinical trial in which half of the test subjects are given the same treatment and everybody else is given a placebo. Only in this case, the test subjects were the places where Philly's most violent crimes were being committed. It was a social scientist's dream, the same kind of real-world laboratory that Rich Mitchell is using to assess the impact of woodland improvement on urban stress in Scotland. Ratcliffe and his colleagues used geographic information system data to identify the 120 most dangerous corners in the city — from 2006 to 2008, the top 5 percent of these corners accounted for 39 percent of all robberies, 42 percent of aggravated assaults and 33 percent of homicides — and then selected 60 to target. Each beat included about 15 intersections and 1.5 miles of roadway. Small patrol zones in places with high population densities, and officers returning to the same street several times each shift, are the keys to effective foot patrols, says Ratcliffe. So is a supportive administration. Commissioner Ramsey and Mayor Michael Nutter were willing to withstand the political fallout of leaving the other five dozen locations less secure.

The three-month experiment took place in the summer of 2009. When factors such as crime displacement were weighed using Thiessen polygons, Voronoi networks and linear regression models (which, to me, qualifies as scientifically robust), targeted corners outperformed the control-group corners by 23 percent. More than 50 violent crimes (homicides, assaults, robberies) were prevented by beat cops, and arrests went up 13 percent. Ratcliffe demonstrated that an intelligence-led approach to foot patrols could indeed cut crime, overturning a long-held mindset among criminologists and other policing experts. More important, it convinced Ramsey to assign every rookie officer to 12 months of foot-patrol duty.

Another criminology experiment, in a rough part of Rotterdam, substantiated both the broken window theory and the ideas of Jane Jacobs. Residents were asked how their community could be improved. Rather than a crackdown on crimes and drugs, they requested cleaner streets, slower traffic and better walkability. After police helped them institute some of these changes, drug crime decreased by 30 percent and burglaries by 22 percent. People had a stronger physical presence, and a greater collective stake, in their neighbourhood.

Although crime reduction was the Philadelphia project's main measure, it also showcased what Ratcliffe calls the ancillary benefits of foot patrol — improved relations between police and the people they serve. This is no small concern in places such as North Philly, where animosity has festered for generations. During the experiment, beat cops stopped pedestrians 64 percent more than their control group co-workers a few blocks away. They searched some but simply talked to others. "It's vital," says Ratcliffe, "to spend time just standing on a street corner, chatting to people, getting a feel for the tempo and rhythm of a place. Within a few weeks, a good foot-patrol officer knows everybody." They know that the drunk on the corner is not a threat because he's always there, but the stranger lurking near the bus stop might be a problem.

"Officers in cars end up perceiving a neighbourhood differently than officers on foot," says Ratcliffe. "If you're in a car, you're only ever exposed to people who are under stress. Either they've been a victim of a crime and you're responding to that crime, or they're a suspect in a crime. Whereas when you're on foot, there's a lot more opportunity to interact with all the normal people in the neighbourhood. People who just by chance or circumstance happen to be living in a poor area or a violent area.

"Crime changes in Philly from block to block, and you only really understand that when you walk from block to block," he says. "Half the people shot in Philly are shot within two blocks of their address. People live and die in very small areas. Foot patrol is an ideal way to understand that microcosm where victims of crime and perpetrators are living out much of their lives."

"Show me what's in your pocket!"

Matt Green was walking past a New York Police Department mobile observation tower — which looks like the runt offspring of one of those lumbering AT-AT snow walkers at the beginning of *The Empire Strikes Back* — when the cop stopped him. A slight, bearded white man in his mid-30s, Green was taking photos with his phone in a predominantly black housing project in the Bronx. He had passed the SkyWatch tower a couple of times already and the white officer was concerned about the bulge in the interloper's back pocket.

"This?" asked Green, reaching behind his right hip, and realizing at that precise moment, as if in slow-motion, when he saw the startled look on the officer's face, that he appeared to be going for a gun.

It was too late to stop. He pulled out a plastic water bottle. Both men exhaled sighs of relief.

The cop's look, Green tells me three weeks later, didn't say, *This guy is going to shoot me.* It was more *Don't tell me I'm going to have to arrest this dumb schmuck.* And *Goddamn paperwork.*

"What are you doing here, anyway?" the officer asked.

Green explained his quest as best he could: a multi-year mission to walk every street of every borough in New York City. Yes, he wants to see and document what's there. But more so, to visit places he has no reason to visit. To tear down all the generalizations of the city and its people that he has absorbed. To submit to a "constant, wide-ranging, uncurated flow of stimulation and information that overwhelms our innate tendency to try to fit everything into a neat and tidy set of preconceptions." Green has no fixed address. He apartment-sits and sleeps on friends' couches, and passively solicits donations online to pay for food and subway tickets. Walking has become a full-time gig. Which is not something one can summarize easily in the 10-second window that New Yorkers usually give to strangers who start talking to them. Typically, he gets blank stares, and then people get edgy, expecting a sales pitch.

"You know, you tell all that to me, I understand," the policeman said that day in the Bronx, after Green gave him a Coles Notes explanation. "But these people" — the officer spread his arms and peered from side to side, even though there was nobody in sight — "you take a picture and they'll kick your ass."

Green has shot thousands of photographs since he started his New York walk on New Year's Day, 2012, and he has been on the receiving end of not a single ass-kicking. Amid countless microcosmic moments, that encounter with a cop was an anomaly. Everyday urban life, whether in the Bronx or North Philly, is rarely dramatic. Walking through a city allows you to appreciate the fine-grained details, the subtle textures, the spontaneous encounters. To leave behind rote apprehension about people you do not know.

It is just before 5 p.m. on a bright, warm Wednesday in East Harlem. I came to New York by train from Philadelphia, and Green and I have been crisscrossing the neighbourhood's brownstone-lined side streets and bustling commercial boulevards on foot since noon. He is wearing cargo shorts, a faded green short-sleeve button-up shirt and brown leather hiking boots — an outfit that has caused passersby to mistake him for a city inspector, an undercover cop and, once, on Staten Island, Crocodile Dundee. On his head is a brown baseball hat embossed with the word *Heddatron*, a surreal play featuring renegade robots and a tormented Henrik Ibsen that was directed by his younger brother, who works in the theatre business in Chicago and is now considered by their parents, retired state government employees in Virginia, to be the son with the normal life.

When he walks around New York all day, which he does three or four days a week, year-round, Green keeps two running tallies: the number of September 11 memorials he sees, both official monuments and homemade tributes, and the number of barbershops that use a Z in place of an S, or a K instead of a C, on their signs. He also watches out for banana vendors, unlocked porta-potties, unusual public art, historic churches, cemeteries, beguiling doorways, imaginative mailboxes, typographic errors on signage and apartment-building standpipes adorned with inventive anti-sitting devices, and he can usually guess, within a few cents, the price of an egg salad sandwich at any of the city's 13,000 bodegas. Green lives on about $15 a day. The cost of his preferred lunch, which he eats without stopping, with lettuce and tomato, and spicy mustard if it's available, typically ranges from $2 to $3.50, depending on the status of the neighbourhood, although $4 is not uncommon in Manhattan. The best deal he can recall is $1.50. His jaw dropped when a deli in Queens charged $5. "That," he declares, "crossed some sort of sandwich threshold."

Green used to have a girlfriend and a respectable career as a transportation engineer. Then the relationship ended and he found it difficult to justify doing a job he didn't enjoy for money he didn't need. Feeling anxious and craving adventure — a textbook case of fugue — he turned his back on five years of highway and roadway design and walked across the United States.

Although he had done a lot of long-distance walking in New York, including a five-day, 150-mile circumnavigation of the city, this was a stretch. Green departed from Rockaway Beach, Queens, in March 2010, wearing a reflective vest and pushing his camping gear in a running stroller, and arrived, five months later, in Rockaway Beach, Oregon. While preparing for the trip, he was bombarded by suggestions that sounded like commands: you *have* to go there, you *need* to see that. Instead, he plotted a direct line to Chicago, to visit his brother, and then west to the Pacific.

Without specific destinations to anticipate, Green could appreciate anything he saw, anywhere he was, instead of counting the miles until he reached, say, South Dakota's Mount Rushmore. "You don't need to know what you're going to see to see interesting things," he says. "That's letting other people's preferences prejudice your reaction. You can just walk across North Dakota. I've driven across places like that and it's incredibly boring. But that generic field at 70 miles per hour is all individual plants at three miles per hour." On his cross-country walk, Green discovered that a blazing yellow sea of canola, lit up by the prairie sun, is a sight to behold.

What's more, the closed-minded, dangerous strangers he was warned about turned out to be welcoming and generous. On dozens of occasions, in small towns and on rural roads, Green was offered a beer, a meal, a bed for the night. His biggest snag was getting away from kind hosts when he had mileage to make. Several times, he was offered lunch just after finishing lunch. "The experiences I had on that walk," he says, "couldn't have been any further from what the media portray America to be."

When he returned to New York, Green's plan to find a job and settle down was no longer palatable. He did some contract work as a health department data collector and spent a few months in the fields of an organic farm in the Hudson Valley. Slowly, his next journey took shape. "I didn't know at the time," he says, "that I would be removing myself so far from mainstream society." And yet, as a sociologist of the streets, he is immersing himself deeply into it. Ultimately, he will cover about 2,500 more miles than William B. Helmreich, a sociology professor who recently walked most blocks in all five boroughs and wrote an ethnographic study called *The New York Nobody Knows*. Waves of immigration and gentrification, argues Helmreich, have fostered a spirit of transformation and optimism. Green makes no such pronouncements. He is simply bearing witness and sharing stories.

When we think about cities, Green says in a TED Talk recorded in Brooklyn, we typically want them to work better for us. To be more productive, livable or engaging. All are important qualities. But if you are trying to make a relationship more enriching and rewarding, you can't focus only on fixing the *other* person, he says. You need to become a better listener, more curious, and to seek out moments of intimacy. New York, like all cities, is complex and bewildering. It's natural to devise labels and rankings to get to know it. To deepen the relationship, though, you could skip the crosstown trip to that trending new restaurant and see what's going on down the block. Or down any block. "Don't try to seek out anything particular, don't even bother trying to draw any conclusions," he says. "Just listen to what the city has to tell you . . . and let your own unique instincts guide you."

On the surface, Green's undertaking is that of a *flâneur*, the literary figure that emerged in 19th-century Paris, a passionate wanderer who studies the city. French poet Charles Baudelaire saw the *flâneur* as a "gentleman stroller of city streets," immersed in the crowd yet a detached observer at the same time, while German philosopher Walter Benjamin considered him a response to the alienation of cities and capitalism. Green's project also speaks to Guy Debord's Situationist concept of a *dérive*, an unplanned drift through an urban landscape. Both of these terms fit within the wider world of psychogeography, a free-spirited investigation of the city, popularized by authors such as Will Self and Shawn Micallef, that incorporates critiques of culture, architecture and urban design, among more playful manifestations. For instance, a walk in which you turn left at the second corner you reach, and then take the next right, repeating the pattern to allow the randomness of the journey to free you from the constraints of time and place that normally dictate our relationship with a city. Yet none of this really encapsulates what Green is doing. Although he plays the role of Baudelaire's detached observer, and alienation is an undercurrent to his walk, Green is mostly looking for those human moments that connect us to the urban web. And there is a scientist's formality to his method. He meticulously maps each day's route in a pocket-sized black notebook, sketching paths through confusing intersections and using cryptic shorthand ("L ACP, R 110") to remind himself where to turn.

Green's fastidiousness and resolve attract press coverage, which generates a small stream of donations. After the *New York Times* published a feature, supporters gave him $8,000, though he doesn't intend to profit. He simply wants to continue his "exhaustive journey through an inexhaustible city" — and, after each outing, to research the day's most compelling images, so he can write the descriptions that accompany the photos on his blog. The documentation, a full-time job itself, is an attempt to assemble a detailed archive of his observations. But the walking, as Henry David Thoreau wrote, is "the enterprise and adventure of the day."

On this day, number 537, we are approaching a dead end on East 117th Street when Green freezes in the middle of the road. "Look!" he gasps, slapping me on the shoulder and pointing toward a barbershop at the base of a refurbished red-brick walk-up. "Krispy Kutz!"

He snaps a photograph of the sleek red-and-black sign with an oversized Z and those glorious K's (it's titled "Barberz #77" on his website, imjustwalkin.com), and then continues heading east. The entire block, not only the building with Krispy Kutz, has been redeveloped. Even Spanish Harlem is gentrifying.

We had just turned off Pleasant Avenue, a legendary mob stronghold where Anthony Salerno, a.k.a. Fat Tony, ran the Genovese crime family. Scenes from *The Godfather* were filmed here. But most evidence of that era is gone. As is any trace, at the terminus of East 117th, of the Washburn Wire Factory, where for more than seven decades workers made springs, piano strings and fences. At one time the largest employer in Manhattan, the factory was shuttered in 1976 and demolished nearly 30 years later. The squatters, addicts and graffiti artists who revelled in the six crumbling structures have been supplanted by the East River Plaza, a 485,000-square-foot vertical big-box mall anchored by Costco and Target.

Green leads me through a Plexiglas-roofed open-air atrium and past the shopping-cart corral to a terrace with a view of Franklin D. Roosevelt Drive and the green waters of the East River. A plaque proclaims our perch to be the Jim Runsdorf Overlook. It's named after a real estate executive who was rowing upstream from this spot on a cold October morning when a motorboat crashed into his racing shell. Runsdorf's body was found by divers three days later. Of course, Green didn't know anything about Runsdorf or Washburn Wire when we happened upon the shopping mall. He rarely knows what he will see. Which, again, is the point of his project.

We climb eight flights of concrete stairs and reach the sun-bleached rooftop deck of the East River Plaza garage, which has space for 1,248 vehicles. There are only a couple of cars, and no people. Green scampers onto a concrete bollard and looks out over the aluminum safety wall. Six lanes of traffic are streaming uptown and downtown along FDR Drive. From above, the sound is soothing, serene. We discuss the possibility of buying a table at Bob's Discount Furniture and a mountain of sandwich meat at Costco, and having one hell of a picnic.

Green points south, to the old mental hospital on Roosevelt Island, where journalist Nellie Bly faked insanity and was committed in 1887, writing an influential exposé on the horrific treatment and conditions faced by patients at the asylum. He looks north to the parkway on-ramp, where an ex-con street artist likes to stand with watermelons and other fruit balanced on his head, or do calisthenics, or set up offbeat installations, such as a stuffed carnival gorilla in a beach chair, demonstrating to drivers the importance of physical health and proper nutrition, or just amusing them as they inch by during rush hour. Green has never actually seen the artist in action, only telltale watermelon rinds and messages tacked onto the surrounding trees. "Otis Houston Jr.," read the first sign that he saw. "Goggle me."

A police boat roars up the East River, sending waves crashing into the shoreline. "I think there's a fuller sense of tranquility when you're out there in the wilderness," Green says, "but you can approach that in the city. This is the urban equivalent of the sea-shore. You get the white noise of traffic. A honk is like an annoying seagull. It's not a disheartening manifestation of humanity.

"People in Manhattan complain about big-box stores coming in, but this is here. They should come and check it out."

Wearing a black *lucha libre* wrestling mask and trailing a shiny black cape, Peatónito steps in front of a silver Jeep Patriot that has nosed into the crosswalk. He places both palms above the front grille, braces his legs, leans in and tries to push the vehicle backward with his bare hands. Sometimes he spray-paints white lines onto the asphalt at intersections where no markings exist. Sometimes he walks across the hoods of cars parked on sidewalks. Sometimes he takes seniors by the hand and helps them cross the street. It can be difficult to navi-gate a megalopolis on foot. *Chilangos* in Mexico City get help from a superhero.

Traffic accidents are a scourge in the Mexican capital. In 2006, nearly 900 pedestrians were killed, and roughly 9.4 of every 100,000 residents die in car crashes each year, well above London (1.9 per 100,000), New York (2.2), Hong Kong (3.8) and Bogotá (4.1). Only Cape Town, South Africa, has meaner streets. Enter Peatónito, whose name means *little pedestrian*. Beneath the mask a political science student and planning consultant named Jorge Cáñez, the *luchador* makes clever street theatre. But his battle cry is real. "The pedestrian is nobody in this city, forgotten by authorities and our own citizenry," he says. "The curious and paradoxical thing is that we are all pedes-trians at some moment. As such, we have forgotten ourselves."

Matt Green and the Philadelphia police have turned to walking to better acquaint themselves with their communities, but they are outliers. Peatónito's performances are more telling. The car rules most of our cities. About 270,000 pedestrians are killed by motor vehicles around the globe every year, according to the World Health Organization. That's 22 percent of the 1.24 million annual traffic deaths. (Road injuries are currently the ninth leading cause of death globally, but the WHO predicts they will soar to third place, behind heart disease and stroke, by 2020.)

More than 47,000 pedestrians were killed on American streets between 2003 and 2012, roughly one-third the number of murder victims. While the annual total has fluctuated around 5,000, the share of traffic fatalities comprised by pedestrians has been slowly creeping up, from 12 to 15 percent. The number of drivers and passengers killed in crashes has been reduced by one-third over the same 10-year span. Improved vehicle design, the enforcement of seat-belt laws and a crackdown on drunk driving are behind this drop, says a national coalition called Smart Growth America. Meanwhile, "we have invested nowhere near the same level of money and energy in providing for the safety and security of people when they are walking." In the U.S., someone is hit by a vehicle while walking every eight minutes. And the risks are not evenly distributed. Seniors, children between the ages of five and nine, racial and ethnic minorities, and residents of lower-income neighbourhoods have a greater chance of ending up in the back of an ambulance.

Google Alert keeps me up to date. Three people were killed on 96th Street in New York's Upper West Side in one week in January 2014, including a doctor who was knocked down by an ambulance and then run over by a sedan, and a nine-year-old boy killed by a taxi while crossing the street with his father. The cabbie got a $300 summons for failing to yield to a pedestrian. In Queens, three teen girls were rushed to hospital after being run down on the sidewalk by an SUV. The driver said he had mistakenly stepped on the gas instead of the brakes. He was not charged.

Distracted driving (talking, texting or tweeting while behind the wheel) is a growing problem. It leads to 1.6 million accidents and 330,000 injuries every year in the U.S., and by 2016, it is expected to cause more traffic fatalities than drunk driving in Canada. But drivers aren't the only culprits. Distracted-walking injuries led to four times as many emergency-room visits in the U.S. in 2012 compared to 2005. For every amusing YouTube video — you know, the woman who tumbled into a shopping-mall fountain in Pennsylvania — there is a chilling counterpoint. A 28-year-old woman, trying to cross a street in downtown Toronto while talking on her phone, marched into the side of a turning truck and was crushed to death under its rear wheels. "Everyone knows to look left and right," says American College of Emergency Physicians spokesperson Dr. Ryan Stanton, who stitches up head lacerations from people walking into stop signs and shin cuts from fire hydrants, "but when you're texting, you forget the rules of survival."

None of this would surprise Siobhan Schabrun, a physical therapist at the University of Western Sydney, in Australia. Her research shows that texting while walking not only distorts the flow of sensory information from your surroundings, it also alters your gait. Essentially, it makes you walk like a robot. Your arms, head and torso move stiffly, and you are more likely to veer out of an intended trajectory, or lose balance if you collide with something. Because your head remains in alignment with your phone, Schabrun suspects that the ear's vestibular system might be receiving "bad information."

Matt Green did not text or talk on his phone while we were together. In fact, he cautioned me that he might have to call for a halt to my questions if there was too much to see. He was tuned in to his surroundings. But the emergence of Peatónito, and this epidemic of pedestrian death and distraction, underscores a sidewalk ballet under siege. To understand how we got here, let's take a closer look at the changes that have shattered the human scale of our lives.

People have long harboured a touch of disdain toward walking. The term *pedestrian*, not in common usage in English until the 18th century, comes from the Latin *pedester*, or *on foot*. It was much sexier to be *equester: on a horse*. The *Oxford English Dictionary* defines pedestrian as "prosaic, plain, commonplace, uninspired (sometimes contrasted with the winged flight of Pegasus)." In other words, Tom Vanderbilt writes in *Traffic*, "not to be on a horse, flying or otherwise, was to be utterly unremarkable and mundane."

As far back as the 14th century BC, nobles in Egypt used horse-drawn chariots to travel from suburban estates with sprawling gardens to the city. Wealthy citizens in ancient Rome also built large villas on the outskirts of town. On a 2,500-year-old clay tablet, Leigh Gallagher writes in *The End of the Suburbs*, a Mesopotamian from the city-state of Ur boasted to the king of Persia that his property "was so close to Babylon that we can enjoy all the advantages of the city, and yet when we come home we are away from all the noise and dust." Cities remained centres of culture and commerce, but in the late 18th and early 19th centuries, the newly rich moved away from the squalid urban centres of industrializing Europe. In 1814, the Fulton Ferry began plying the East River between Manhattan and Brooklyn, and Brooklyn Heights became the world's first large-scale commuter suburb. Americans took this exodus to a new level after Henry Ford unveiled the Model-T in 1908. Car culture and suburban growth exploded after World War II. Automobiles signalled affluence and independence. Leaping over the boundaries of time and space, we were smitten.

In North America, metropolitan areas mushroomed as developers built single-land-use subdivisions of cookie-cutter tract houses and planners supplied freeways and shopping malls to streamline travel and the consumption of lawnmowers and patio furniture. This car-centric landscape changed our lives, and a handful of recessionary speed bumps did little to slow its advance. Three-quarters of U.S. residential construction between 1980 and 2010 was in the suburbs, even though the reasons we fled downtown — sewage, smoke, disease — were no longer pressing.

Fuelled by cheap gasoline and subsidized by the state through preferential taxation and credit schemes, these "dispersed cities" were a capitalist's dream, Charles Montgomery writes in *Happy City: Transforming Our Lives Through Urban Design*. Private automobiles carried people to private space. Touting safety and freedom for drivers, the automobile lobby convinced Americans that pedestrians had to be controlled. Jaywalking became a crime. Cities ripped out streetcar and train tracks. "Our national flower," said American architecture critic Lewis Mumford, "is the concrete cloverleaf."

Much has been written about the consequences of suburbanization: homogeneity, as fixed price points and racial discrimination discouraged mixing; severed inner cities, as highways feeding downtown were pushed through working-class districts; and a reliance on the car for daily activities, heightening our dependence on petroleum products and fostering unprecedented levels of physical inactivity. The suburb, Montgomery writes, "is the most expensive, resource-intense, land-gobbling, polluting way of living ever built." Home to half the planet's population, cities consume 75 percent of the world's energy and produce 80 percent of greenhouse-gas emissions. Suburbanites emit twice as much carbon as people who live downtown.

There are also health considerations. In Toronto, rates of diabetes among baby boomers are higher in the suburbs than in the city core, despite the relative affluence of the suburbs, a geographical determinant that generally presages health indicators. The stats are reversed because downtown dwellers walk more.

Torontonians have the longest average work commute in Canada: about 33 minutes each way, on par with New York and Washington, D.C. Almost 90 percent of Americans drive to work every day, and more than 75 percent drive to work alone. (In Canada and the U.K., roughly three-quarters and two-thirds of people commute by car, respectively.) Montgomery cites studies that conclude that the farther people commute, the less happy they are, and not just when they're stuck in traffic, but with their lives in general. An extra 23 minutes of commuting has the same effect on happiness as a 19 percent reduction in income, Swiss economists Alois Stutzer and Bruno Frey write in a paper titled "Stress That Doesn't Pay." Someone with a 60-minute commute has to earn 40 percent more than someone who walked to work to be as satisfied with their life.

Harvard political scientist Robert Putnam looked into the social impact of commuting in his book *Bowling Alone: The Collapse and Revival of American Community*. Turns out, the amount of time we spend driving to and from work is a determinant of civic engagement. "Each 10 additional minutes in daily commuting time," he writes, "cuts involvement in community affairs by 10 percent — fewer public meetings attended, fewer committees chaired, fewer petitions signed, fewer church services attended, and so on." If you leave home at dawn, fight traffic en route to the office and do the same thing on the way back, you are tense and tired, and may not have anything left to give.

When the 1970s rolled around, one in ten Americans walked to work. Today, fewer than one in 40 do. French philosopher Bernard-Henri Lévy calls this auto-heavy lifestyle a "global, total obesity that spares no realm of life, public or private. An entire society that, from the top down, from one end to the other, seems prey to this obscure derangement that slowly causes an organism to swell, overflow, explode."

Montgomery opens his narrative by describing the revolutionary tenure of Enrique Peñalosa, mayor of Bogotá, Colombia, from 1998 to 2001. Peñalosa kick-started the transformation of one of the world's most dangerous and polluted cities into a safer, happier place by turning gridlocked roads into avenues for cyclists and improving the transit system, and by investing in parks and other public spaces. This made it easier for impoverished residents to travel around their city, and gave them somewhere to socialize, without taking anything away from wealthier citizens. In fact, it simplified their travel, too, by reducing roadway congestion.

Money, as Montgomery shows, does not buy happiness. Household wealth soared in the U.S., U.K. and Canada until the 2008 recession, but surveys do not reveal a corresponding spike in well-being. Only that we had more cars and larger homes, and produced more garbage. "What are our needs for happiness?" asks Peñalosa. To be around other people. Contact with nature. To feel some sort of equality. And, he says, "we need to walk, just as birds need to fly."

The pendulum is starting to swing back. In 2011, urban population growth in the United States outpaced suburban growth — an inversion not seen since the advent of the automobile. To millions of boomers, families and millennials, the most desirable neighbourhoods are dense, central and full of eyes on the street. Walkability is poised for a comeback.

Jane Jacobs died in 2006, but the movement she championed is stronger than ever. In the 1960s, she led protest campaigns that stopped construction of the Lower Manhattan Expressway (which would have destroyed Washington Square Park) and the extension of Toronto's Spadina Expressway. These were controversial fights. But grouped under the umbrella of "new urbanism," her ideas are now seen as rational, not radical, by hundreds of big-city mayors, from New York's Bill de Blasio to Calgary's Naheed Nenshi.

In Canada's oil capital, Nenshi has made public transit and multi-use paths one of the cornerstones of his mandate. Immediately after being re-elected, in 2013, he pushed ahead with a downtown bike lane and vowed to eliminate the $4,800 "sprawl subsidy" that every new suburban house receives. (New communities require significant infrastructure, from roads and water pipes to schools and libraries. Developers cover 78 percent of the costs in Calgary, while taxpayers foot the rest of the bill, which reached $33 million in 2012.)

Just one month after taking office, in January 2014, de Blasio put pedestrian safety at the top of his agenda. After that deadly week on 96th Street in the Upper West Side, he proposed a citywide speed limit of 25 miles per hour, down from the current 30, and stronger enforcement. Drivers speeding or failing to yield cause 70 percent of New York's pedestrian fatalities. Sixty-three percent of the pedestrians who died in the U.S. between 2003 and 2012 were killed on roads with a speed limit of 40 mph or faster. In June 2014, de Blasio signed into law a spate of new traffic bills. The speed limit will indeed drop to 25 mph, dozens of new 20 mph slow zones near schools will be created each year, cabbies responsible for crashes that kill or critically injury somebody will lose their licence and failing to yield to a pedestrian with the right-of-way will become a criminal misdemeanour. "Death and injury on city streets is not acceptable," said the mayor, "and we will no longer regard serious crashes as inevitable."

New York's new laws are based on Sweden's Vision Zero Initiative. In many ways, Scandinavia is at the forefront of the urbanist movement. Internationally renowned Danish architect and urban designer Jan Gehl was an early adopter of Jacobs' vision. Gehl has infused his practice with sociology and psychology — the human side of architecture, all too frequently steamrolled in the quest for progress. He pushes for incremental change, such as Copenhagen's 40-year-long evolution from car-saturated cacophony into a bicycling and pedestrian poster child. In 1962, when the central retail street Strøget became a car-free zone, skeptics said the city was too far north for the experiment to work. Foot traffic jumped 35 percent in the first year alone, and Strøget has grown into Europe's longest pedestrian shopping area, drawing 250,000 people every day in the summer and nearly half that in winter. "A good city is like a good party," says Gehl. "You know it's working when people stay for much longer than really necessary, because they are enjoying themselves."

American city planner Jeff Speck has also stepped into Jacobs' shoes. In *Walkable City: How Downtown Can Save America, One Step at a Time*, he serves up example after compelling example of communities taking concrete measures to reimagine their futures. The book is a call to arms, arguing that urban walkability is not high-minded idealism, but a simple, practical solution to a range of complex problems, including economic competitiveness, public welfare and environmental sustainability. It is a counter-strike against the "fattened roads, emaciated sidewalks, deleted trees, fry-pit drive-thrus and ten-acre parking lots" that have made pedestrian travel "a mere theoretical possibility" in many cities.

In Los Angeles a few years back, I booked a motel kitty-corner from Universal Studios' CityWalk theme park, where I would be reporting on a story for a week. Even though there was only one main intersection between my musty room and my daily destination, I needed about 20 minutes to reach CityWalk, an expedition that took me under a freeway, across a wide, fast-moving boulevard, up a busy access road and through a series of parking lots. All to reach a three-block-long replica streetscape flanked by chain restaurants. (To be fair, L.A. is improving. Inspired by Bogotá, regular events shut streets to cars and draw thousands of cyclists, rollerbladers and walkers. Although when writer David Hochman invited a couple of friends to join him, they showed up late because they left one car at the finish line and drove another to the starting point. "People, this is Los Angeles," he felt like telling them. "You only need one car for a pedestrian-friendly outing.")

Walkability has many social rewards, writes Speck, chief among them urban vitality. Meccas such as New York and San Francisco know this and are on the right track, but elsewhere, city engineers and planners have long been distracted by what he calls the twin gods of Smooth Traffic and Ample Parking, converting city cores into "places that are easy to get to and not worth arriving at." In the 1980s, urban beautification schemes in North America focused on the five B's: bricks, banners, bandstands, bollards and berms. These features "now grace many an abandoned downtown." In the 1960s and 1970s, more than 150 main streets across the U.S. were pedestrianized — and dozens failed immediately. According to Speck's General Theory of Walkability, nurturing the "fragile species" that we know as the pedestrian requires walking routes that meet four main criteria. They have to be *useful*, taking us to the places we need to be regularly. They must be *safe*, which means not only protected from cars, but also from other threats. They should be *comfortable* — i.e., not a windswept streetscape dominated by monolithic office towers and parking lots. And they should be *interesting*, sidewalks "lined by unique buildings with friendly faces [where] signs of humanity abound."

Thankfully, there's a demographic migration afoot. Empty-nest baby boomers find themselves craving the cultural activities and easy movement an urban core can provide. Their large suburban homes are expensive to heat and maintain, says Brookings Institution economist Christopher Leinberger, and their neighbourhoods feel iso-lating, especially because aging makes driving more difficult. There are nearly 80 million boomers in the U.S., a quarter of the population. Their housing and lifestyle decisions will make waves. Meanwhile, millennials born in the 1980s and 1990s are an even larger cohort, and they are falling out of love with the car. Since the 1990s, the percentage of miles driven by 20-somethings in the U.S. has fallen from 20.8 to 13.7, and since the 1970s, the number of 19-year-olds choosing not to get a driver's licence has jumped from 8 to 23 percent.

Walkable City is full of nuggets like this. Nearly two-thirds of college-educated millennials choose where they want to live before looking for a job, notes Speck, and 77 percent plan to live in America's urban cores. This demand represents an opportunity for the real-estate and building industries that could lay the foundation for North America's economy for decades, just as the construction of far-flung subdivisions (and the roads that took us there) did in the 1950s and 1960s. Speck compares this migration to our television-viewing habits. In the 1970s, sitcoms such as *The Brady Brunch* showcased the suburban ideal — detached homes on leafy lots — while cop shows like *Hawaii 5-0* linked downtown to crime. Skip forward a couple of decades, and the airwaves were dominated by *Friends* and *Seinfeld*. Suddenly, the big city was not only safe, it was cool.

Mercer, a global consulting firm, conducts an annual quality-of-living survey, ranking cities around the world based on 10 categories, including their social, economic, cultural and natural environments. In 2012, as usual, Vienna and Zurich topped the list, followed by Auckland, Munich and Vancouver. Europe, Australia, New Zealand and Canada dominated the next 20 positions (Ottawa was 14th), and the first American city was Honolulu. Only eight cities in the U.S., including San Francisco, New York, Washington and Boston, are in the top 50. Speck compares these rankings to the walkability of American cities and isn't surprised that sprawling metropolitan areas like Los Angeles and Houston don't make the grade. Mercer's top cities, year after year, are places "that are better for walking than driving."

The bulk of *Walkable City* is a 10-step primer on how to make communities more pedestrian-friendly. It should be required reading for every urban planner. Every politician too. And, well, anybody who spends time in the city.

First up, recommends Speck, put cars in their place. The second-class-citizen treatment of pedestrians, he believes, is not an inevitability. While other metropolitan areas were sprawling, Washington, D.C., received just 10 of a proposed 450 miles of interstate highway, thanks to loud and determined resistance. ("White men's roads through black men's homes" was one of the protest slogans.) Money and space were instead allocated to the expansive Metrorail system, a decision that reverberates through the lively, prosperous urban core.

Speck doesn't call for the elimination of cars from our cities. We don't all live in Copenhagen. "The key," he writes, "is to welcome cars in the proper number and at the proper speed." Which leads to the second of his suggestions: mix the uses. Although zoning codes were responsible for separating smoke-spewing factories from the places where we live and play, these laws have led to a separation of our homes from just about everything else we do in a city. Make it easier to "work, shop, eat, drink, learn, recreate, convene, worship, heal, visit, celebrate, sleep" by making the places we do these things within walking distance of each other, he says — introduce zoning codes and development plans that encourage a diverse range of land-use options within the city core. This impacts not only transportation and happiness, but also safety, says Gehl. A variety of uses can lead to around-the-clock activity on a street, even if it's just light from residential windows brightening an empty road, "a comforting signal that people are nearby."

Mixing the uses also speaks to the Dutch concept of *woonerf*, a shared street on which pedestrians and cyclists have legal priority. There are often no barriers separating these modes of travel from cars, no curbs or fences, but driving speed is restricted to a walking pace and accident stats are always much lower than on regular streets. When collisions do occur, injuries are far less severe because of the reduced speed.

Speck's third step, get the parking right, notes that there are roughly 750 million parking spaces in America, covering more urban acres than any other land use. These rectangles of asphalt cost anywhere from $4,000 to $40,000 apiece to build, depending on the value of the land they are on and whether they are on the surface or in a parking garage. This oversupply effectively provides a massive subsidy to drivers, "which in turn undermines the quality of walking, biking, and transit." With 250 million cars on American's roads, more than half a billion spaces are empty much of the time. Why so many? Because of rules that stipulate the number of parking spots in each new development, from gas stations to malls and swimming pools — one space per 2,500 gallons of water — and because of the bureaucratic fight required to override these rules, even for projects built at transit hubs or in pedestrian-oriented neighbourhoods.

Donald Shoup, a professor of urban planning at the University of California, Los Angeles, and the author of *The High Cost of Free Parking*, recommends that American cities adopt a more European approach: instead of requiring parking and limited density, they should limit parking and require density. He also suggests raising the rates at street-side parking meters, which are generally around one-quarter the price of nearby off-street parking lots, leading to instances in which, according to one study in Manhattan, one-third of all traffic congestion was made up of cars circling to find somewhere to park. A friend who moved to Ottawa from Manhattan says it wasn't uncommon to spend an hour trolling around his apartment for parking. Eventually, he would give up and phone his wife, who would meet him at the base of the building, take over the wheel and continue the hunt.

Contrary to conventional thinking, paid street parking doesn't drive people away from downtown, says Shoup; it fosters turnover, something merchants relish. More customers, more sales. Although it is often dangerous to cyclists, curb-lane parking makes sidewalks safer for pedestrians, creating a buffer between foot traffic and speeding cars. And the money municipalities make from their meters can be put toward improving sidewalks and lighting, and adding trees and street furniture, making central shopping and entertainment districts that are much more pleasant.

Number four on Speck's list: design efficient, integrated, nodal transit networks. People like to walk to the bus or train, and then to their destination. Five: protect the pedestrian with small blocks, and streets with fewer, narrower lanes. Small blocks give pedestrians more choices and shorten most walking trips, and are the variable most predictive of injury and death in car accidents, University of Connecticut engineers concluded after studying more than 130,000 crashes. The smaller the block, the smaller the streets around it, the slower cars move, with "a doubling of block size [leading to] a tripling of fatalities." (Streets that have been narrowed, by the way, tend not to lose vehicle capacity, just as widening streets rarely reduces congestion, thanks to the phenomenon of "induced demand" — when the supply of something, like roads, is increased, people use it even more.)

I will share one more of Speck's recommendations: shape the spaces. Humans evolved to need "prospect and refuge," he writes — places like the forest edge, which offered both somewhere to hide and an open escape route. This is why we typically don't like massive surface parking lots or tower-in-the-park residential enclaves.

In one of the first research projects of its kind, planning consultant Jane Farrow and University of Toronto geography professor Paul Hess analyzed the walkability of Toronto's high-rise neighbourhoods. They found that the majority of residents are carless and depend on walking and transit. That many of these neighbourhoods were built after World War II, with the assumption that apartment dwellers would have cars, creating environments that funnel pedestrians onto wide, high-speed arterial roads. That vulnerable groups, including children, women and the elderly, are fearful of walking, especially at night. That persistent concerns — pooling water, broken benches, poor lighting, missing curb cuts, icy sidewalks, overflowing garbage bins — contribute to feelings of disenfranchisement and resignation, which in turn make maintenance and repairs less likely. And that despite these shortcomings, people enjoy walking in their neighbourhoods because it fosters connections to their community. "Walking environments are not simply routes from A to B," write Hess and Farrow. "They are connective tissue where critical social interactions can occur that knit people together."

Some interactions tear people apart. The aggression and threat of violence that women experience while walking, especially at night, is a gender disparity that cannot be solved through city planning or policy change. Harassment and assault, or the risk thereof, limit the right of equal access to public space. Solnit devotes a chapter to this subject in *Wanderlust*. "Women's walking is often construed as performance rather than transport," she writes, "with the implication that women walk not to see but to be seen . . . which means that they are asking for whatever attention they receive." A video that went viral in 2014 documented an actress getting propositioned and cat-called more than 100 times in ten hours as she walked the streets of New York City. A 2012 American survey found that nearly half of all women are afraid of walking alone at night in their own neighbourhoods, more than double the rate reported by men. Despite a growing awareness about violence against women and rape culture, addressing this inequality will require a movement much deeper than any urban makeover.

By the end of his New York odyssey, Matt Green will have covered nearly 9,000 miles.

"Do you ever get bored while walking?" I ask.

Some parts of the city, such as Harlem, are more lively than quieter, suburban places, like Long Island, he concedes. "But this walk has made me think about what boredom means. Nobody asked me that question when I was an engineer and I sat in a cubicle, under fluorescent lights, doing pretty much the same thing all day every day. Out here, it's always something new."

Below 125th Street, the main east-west strip in Harlem, on Adam Clayton Powell Jr. Boulevard, named after the first New Yorker with African-American roots elected to Congress, Green snaps a photo of a squiggly pedestrian-crossing icon with a scannable QR code. The code takes you to the website of an art project called Curbside Haiku, sponsored by the city's Department of Transportation. In this case, it's a poem by John Morse:

> Imagine a world
> Where your every move matters
> Welcome to that world

We pause in the busy plaza below the Adam Clayton Powell Jr. State Office Building. It's the tallest structure in Harlem, and at its base is the kind of public space that Speck would love. The sunny square is packed. There is a health fair going on, with massages, dental work and medical consultations being offered for free under white tents.

As the afternoon drifts on, Green points out a rocky outcrop near Morningside Park and gives me a lesson in the geology of Manhattan. We eat juicy black mulberries off a lush tree across the street from a boarded-up department store, and he rhymes off a list of wild fruits and weeds that he snacks on while walking. Figs, persimmons, lamb's quarter. There's an amazing raspberry patch in Queens, and a vine of concord grapes on a pedestrian bridge over the Bronx Expressway. "During the summer," he says, "I could survive on what I find growing beside the road."

Then we get to East 117th Street and he spots the Krispy Kutz. And then we are on top of the East River Plaza parkade, soothed by the river and FDR Drive. And then it's time to get moving.

We descend eight flights of stairs — "I kinda consider elevators and escalators to be cheating," says Green — and see a burly man with a beard and a ponytail using a razor blade to scrape white paint off the windshield of a 1965 Ford Mustang. The car, everything except its tires painted white, is parked behind the open hatch of a semi-truck in the curb lane of the street beside the mall. Instead of racing stripes, it is adorned with parallel six-inch-wide strips of black cornrowed hair, from front grille to back bumper.

The guy with the ponytail notices us staring. He shrugs, smiles sheepishly and half says, half asks — rhyming with *naught* — "art."

In fact, it's called "American Hero #4," explains artist Hugh Hayden, who emerges from the parkade, takes the razor blade and enlarges the porthole in his acrylic and synthetic-hair installation, which trucker Mike Tobey has just driven back from an exhibition in Pittsburgh. "The cornrows represent African-American identity," says Hayden, a young black man with thick-rimmed glasses, "and the car is classic Americana."

The four of us start talking. Green explains his project and the two men instantly get it. "My father and I were going to do the same thing," says Tobey, "but in a car."

Hayden drives away slowly, cautiously, as if peering through an icy windshield. Tobey fires up his truck. Green and I walk on. "That was a quintessential New York scene," he says. "It was awesome. I spend the majority of my time in places that people don't think of as New York, which is funny, because they make up the majority of the city."

Gunpoint robberies. Rapes. Crack deals. PCP addicts with superhuman strength. Cops aren't easily surprised in North Philly. But right now, officers Brian Nolan and Mike Farrell are stumped.

They're staring through a chain-link fence at the corner of Montgomery Avenue and 27th Street, about a dozen blocks from the intersection where Moses Walker, Jr., was killed. A small brown horse is placidly munching on thorn bushes in an overgrown yard.

"I think it's legal to keep a horse in the city," says Farrell, looking up and down the block for clues. "It has something to do with the square footage of the property."

"You see everything on these streets," mutters Nolan.

"Have you ever seen a horse here before?" I ask.

"No."

Two grandmothers in floral-print church dresses and wide-brimmed matching hats stop and peer through the fence.

"What's that?"

"Horse," Nolan says matter-of-factly.

"Is he a good horse?"

"I don't know, ma'am. I just met him."

"Happy Father's Day, y'all," the women say before walking away.

Farrell knocks on the door of the house beside the yard. No answer. Nolan pushes a handful of grass through the fence. The horse steps toward him, then lowers its head to drink out of a bucket of weedy water.

A man in a bright orange shirt, a large gold chain dangling from his neck, approaches and introduces himself as Mr. Pick. "What's goin' on?" he asks.

Nolan explains that they're concerned about whether the horse has enough food and water. And why it's there. They may call the SPCA.

"No, everything's aiight," says Mr. Pick. "The horse belongs to a guy who lives down the street. This is his momma's house. The horse was just put in here this morning.

"Ain't nobody just dump the horse here," he adds. "It's used to give kids pony rides and stuff like that."

Mr. Pick assures the officers that the animal will be cared for and waves goodbye with a folded newspaper. "Happy Father's Day," he says while crossing the street.

Because of all of the block parties, because of the drinking, because of the heat, because it is Saturday, because this is the 22nd District, Nolan and Farrell keep promising that I'll see some "action." Crowds plus alcohol equals arguments; then the guns come out. There have been five shootings in the last two weeks. That's typical. But as we crisscross the neighbourhood, it's dog-day quiet. Nolan and Farrell pass the time by exchanging Father's Day greetings with men washing cars and playing cards. It's now 4 p.m., two hours until their shift ends; I wouldn't be surprised to see tumbleweeds rolling down the road.

And then their radios burst to life.

Somebody has been shot in the thigh near a bar called Sara's Place, 20 blocks away. Nolan and Farrell set a fast clip, but after a couple of minutes we hop into the back of a cruiser that's speeding to the scene. "So far, all we know is that a guy got shot," a gruff plainclothes detective announces when we arrive, nodding toward a bullet casing on the road. "And, of course, nobody saw nothing."

Nolan and Farrell are ordered to help cordon off the intersection with yellow police tape. The detective asks who I am, then tells me to stay out of the way. A young female officer unspooling tape asks who I am, then tells me to stay out of way.

I retreat to a wall beneath the awning of a corner store across the street from Sara's Place. A man holding hands with a little girl in a pink dress asks me what happened.

"Somebody got shot in the thigh."

"Aw, is that all," he says, ducking under the tape and continuing along the sidewalk.

A teenager wearing a backwards ball cap approaches and asks the female cop what happened, then looks her up and down. "You look beautiful, ma'am."

"I try."

"You don't have to try, baby. Just keep doing what you're doing."

"Uh-huh."

"What's your name, baby?"

"Officer Bell."

"Nah, what's your first name?"

"Officer."

As two dozen cops comb the area for clues, I start talking to Carlton Addison, a war veteran who tells me he walks this stretch of 29th Street every day for exercise, "to keep the old limbs moving."

"I was in Vietnam," he says. "Here is more dangerous."

Addison moved to Philadephia a year ago, from New York, to be close to his mother. Already, he has seen half a dozen people jumped on the street, and too many robberies to count, especially around the start of the month, when social-security cheques arrive. Addison has been robbed twice since coming to Philly. Now he carries a gun. That, and seeing more cops on the street, helps him feel safe. But mostly, he says, it's the gun. "I'm not going to be a victim a third time."

Father's Day. I'm heading back to the 22nd District for another tag-along shift. My hotel, located amid the stylish restaurants and boutiques of the historic Rittenhouse Square neighbourhood, is on the same street as the police station, just two miles away.

The tree canopy, cafés and white faces thin out as I walk due north. Over the Vine Street Expressway and past Fairmount Avenue, barbed wire tops fences and radios carry out of open windows. "Turn in your unwanted guns, get a $100 ShopRite card," a DJ on Old School 100.3 announces. "Help end gun violence." A police car idles in the shade down an alley.

The sidewalk is cracked, but sparrows chirp from the branches of saplings, and strangers say hello. A pastor sweeping the steps of his church, a postie on the job despite the Sabbath. Jay, smoking a roach on the stoop of his century-old brownstone, sparks up a conversation. He has lived here for all of his 56 years. The neighbourhood is rough, he says, but it's starting to change. Developers are renovating and building new homes to rent to Temple students. The police presence helps, says Jay. "People don't give cops the credit they should get. It's a salvage job. They doing the best they can. And things be more personal when you walking." Then Jay tells me about his own salvage job: he wants to start a trash-removal business. A contract from the university would give him a solid start. "The dean of Temple, he gotta get with me. Who else is gonna clean up this shit? Mr. Sweepy, that's who!"

At HQ, I put on another flak jacket and meet my new partners: James Walls, 27, and Jeffrey Lavar, 24. Both graduated from police academy in March and have been on the job for three months. Lavar, tall and thin, always wanted to be a cop. Walls, average height with a stocky build, spent four years in the U.S. Navy before police academy.

Lavar and Walls are black, but they don't think that matters in North Philly. "All people see," says Walls, "is the blue shirt."

Although we walk different streets, today is a carbon copy of my shift with Nolan and Farrell. Banter with grandmothers, shooting hoops with kids, hard glares from hard men. Earsplitting hip hop pulses from a stack of speakers in a park. Men drink out of paper bags. Lavar and Walls don't look up as they pass. At 2 p.m., we return to HQ for a Father's Day barbecue.

Sgt. Bisarat Worede sets me up with a burger and some potato salad, then turns his attention back to the dozen officers on break. They are teasing and boasting, and complaining about paperwork. Typewriters are still used to fill out certain forms in the 22nd District. Some young cops have never used — or seen — a typewriter before. "It's the economy," Worede says. "We could get more computers, but that would mean fewer officers on the street. The economy is the biggest issue we have around here." Poverty, unemployment, a lack of opportunity: there is a limit to what the police can do. "Why put a band-aid," he asks, "on a wound that really needs stitches?"

In Chicago, which led American cities with more than 500 homicides in 2012, extra foot beats in high-crime zones were a central part of police superintendent Garry McCarthy's response to the killings. The rash of murders made headlines around the country — a 15-year-old honour student named Hadiya Pendleton was gunned near President Barack Obama's house, drawing the president to the city, where he addressed the out-of-control gang violence in a fiery speech. McCarthy's Operation Impact, which is similar to a strategy he helped implement while with the NYPD, has been effective. There were 415 homicides in Chicago in 2013. Other measures, such as a summer jobs program that employed 20,000 young people, have also played a big role. "Not one of those kids was affected by gun violence this summer," said Mayor Rahm Emanuel, "and I don't believe for a minute that if they didn't have jobs they would be safe."

After lunch, the radios carried by Walls and Lavar are virtually silent. The cookouts are still going on, but the only commotion occurs when the officers are heckled by a group of men who are trying to coax them into the park for a beer or some ribs.

"Pretty quiet," yawns Lavar. "Everybody is just chillin'."

"Or in church," says Walls.

Last night was different.

After the shooting, when Nolan and Farrell went off duty, I rode around in a cruiser until 2 a.m. with another pair of officers, veterans Chris Toman and Ray D'Amico. I wanted to see the difference between walking and driving. The contrast was jarring, like being bounced around on the hard plastic back seat as we raced between domestic disputes, gun calls and arguments outside house parties.

Toman floored it if there was a sense of urgency, several times with a police chopper overhead. On some streets, dozens of people stood around in the dark, drinking and talking loudly. Lads up to no good? Or friends and neighbours letting off some steam? Cars squealing to a stop, red and blue lights flashing, it didn't matter. The police were intruders, there to enforce somebody else's law.

At midnight, Toman and D'Amico responded to a car fire. About 100 people were watching, pointing, hollering. The atmosphere was festive, with an edge. Moving bystanders down the block, Toman told me that people often torch abandoned vehicles for cheap entertainment.

The flames were ten feet high when a fire engine pulled up. The crowd cheered. "Everybody loves the fire department," said Toman, "but they hate us. The firemen come to help, and we put people in jail."

"That's the job I really wanted," said D'Amico, "but they weren't hiring."

four

ECONOMY

"In exchange for profit and speed, we are losing the ability to make someone feel special. . . . While technology has vastly improved our lives in some ways, it has taken the humanity out of being a human."

— *Melanie Mackenzie*, The Coast

"All the fancy economic development strategies, such as developing a biomedical cluster, an aerospace cluster, or whatever the current economic development 'flavour of the month' might be, do not hold a candle to the power of a great walkable urban place."

— *Christopher Leinberger*, The Option of Urbanism: Investing in a New American Dream

Christine Murray pulls up beside the curb on a leafy dead-end street. She steps out of her Ford Transit Connect, a compact white van with an aardvark nose and a stylish red swoosh that runs the length of the vehicle. Murray swings open the rear doors and slides a couple dozen bundles of letters, flyers and magazines into a dual satchel, then heaves the bag onto her back and cinches the padded harness around her shoulders and waist. Wearing knobby grey hiking shoes, she sets off briskly along Parkview Road, navigating the front paths and porch steps of tidy bungalows and boxy duplexes without looking down. Her feet know the route.

Murray, 48, has been a Canada Post "delivery agent" in Ottawa for 12 years. The official corporate designation sounds better than "mailwoman," at least, and "letter carrier" no longer does the job justice. Murray is five-foot-three and weighs 100 pounds. The maximum allowable weight of her bag is 35 pounds, and she must be able to carry parcels of up to 50 pounds. The load is manageable, although she has monthly appointments with a massage therapist and a chiropractor. She also visits an Active Release Techniques practitioner, who exerts hand pressure to break up the fibrous bands that form in the soft tissues of the muscles in her legs, which log around ten miles each shift.

But the biggest pain, Murray tells me as she shortcuts through gaps between hedges, is that every task she has to perform is assigned a "time value." From the start of her workday at the Station C distribution centre, where she sequences her allotment of correspondence and solicitations in large grey plastic bins, to carting those bins to the van and driving to her route, to actually delivering the mail, and then driving to the next stopping point to hit another couple of blocks, every move she makes has been quantified. Each lift and step is supposed to take a prescribed number of seconds. There is no accounting for a short chat with an elderly shut-in or a quick game of fetch with a friendly dog. A pair of border collies used to wait for Murray to throw their chew toys. "I think it was something we both needed," she says, "but I don't have time for that anymore."

When I walk my daughters home from school, the postman who serves our neighbourhood always stops to talk. The girls race ahead to greet Gilles. "I've got a package from Grandma," he'll say with a wink. Or, "Your cat magazine is here." Once, he attended to and called an ambulance for a neighbour who had fallen and cut himself badly, and he regularly helps people move couches or lift canoes onto the roofs of cars. As innocent as these encounters are, Gilles is going rogue.

The mailman's steady presence on our street is reassuring — a "benign symbol of the larger web of governance," proclaims the *New York Times*, and "of the national community as a whole." As pen-named postie Bill Walker wrote in an essay for the *Walrus*, "[L]ike the firefighter and the crossing guard, the letter carrier is one of the uniformed characters that help ground kids in a world they don't wholly understand." A world that is changing fast.

In 2008, Canada Post unveiled its ambitious Postal Transformation strategy, a $2-billion undertaking that included recalibrated time values and the purchase of hundreds of those zippy white vans. The crown corporation was under pressure to streamline and modernize its operations. The change was overdue, yet things didn't exactly work out. The new time values, says Murray, were calculated by managers who had never delivered mail. Strains and other injuries spiked among letter carriers, their union protested. And the strategy's main goal — financial stability — remains elusive.

"Our role is evolving," Murray said during the day we spent together, "to the point where we'll probably disappear. Door-to-door delivery is going to vanish. Give it a few years."

Less than a month later, Canada Post swung the axe. It announced that urban home delivery will be phased out over a five-year period, eliminating up to 8,000 jobs. Most of those workers will leave by attrition (thousands are expected to retire), and only about one-third of Canada's 15.3 million households receive mail at the door; the rest already retrieve letters and junk mail from community boxes. Outwardly, then, the decision is prudent. Facing a 25-percent decrease in mail volume between 2008 and 2013, and a projected drop of 25 percent in the next five years, Canada Post would be looking at an annual deficit of $1 billion by 2020, according to the Conference Board of Canada. Something had to be done.

But wait. The corporation made a profit in 17 of the 18 years leading up to its 2013 announcement, including a record surplus of $443 million in 2010. The parcel business is booming, fed by e-commerce. Meanwhile, the United States Postal Service, a massive federal entity in that bastion of capitalism, earned $67.3 billion U.S. in 2012 and maintains a workforce of more than 500,000, including almost 8,000 letter carriers who deliver mail entirely on foot, the legendary USPS Fleet of Feet. And in the U.K., Royal Mail posted a pre-tax profit of £363 million in fiscal 2013–2014, albeit as a newly privatized company, a change ushered in by chief executive Moya Greene, who had previously served as the CEO of Canada Post. (Defending the service cuts in this country, current chief executive Deepak Chopra told the House of Commons that regular walks to the community mailbox will be good for seniors — not a bad idea for those who are able.)

I wanted to spend a shift with a postie because they walk all day. Are people who do this for a living, I wondered, happier or healthier than the rest of us? If so, what insights can they share? And: are they hiring? The labour climate at Canada Post waylaid those questions, as well as my desire to don the uniform. It could have been a good fit, but even before the end of home delivery made headlines, Murray advised me to look elsewhere.

What I saw were bigger tremors. A global pyramid scheme that's starting to sway. Despite our appetite for online shopping, an institution that dates back to Confederation felt it had to eliminate its core service to survive. Information moves at a breakneck pace, and Canada Post's delivery agents could not keep up, casualties of an economy driven by cheap fuel, quick returns and an insatiable thirst for growth. Businesses must adapt or they will die. But is speed the only answer? Can slowing down also pay off?

Amazon.com is the world's largest online retailer. It had revenues of $74 billion U.S. in 2013 and is selling perishable groceries in select American cities in addition to its regular stock of books, electronics, inflatable furniture, diapers, Halloween costumes for dogs, zombie brain Jell-O moulds, sex toys and every other conceivable product, plus many you can't even imagine. (Sigmund Freud action figure, anybody?) The company wants to use drones to make deliveries. There are rumours that robots will soon take over its distribution centres. But for now, because of the sheer variety of merchandise carried by Amazon, and the organizational jumble on its shelves, whenever you proceed through the checkout from the comfort of home, a human "picker" in a warehouse the size of several football fields gets his or her marching orders. We are outsourcing our walking with single-click shopping.

Pickers cover roughly 7 to 15 miles a day on foot. Handheld sat nav units tell them which aisle and shelf to go to, and count down the seconds they have been allotted to get there. The devices also help supervisors keep track of the pickers' productivity. "You're sort of like a robot, but in human form," an Amazon manager explained to the *Financial Times*. "It's human automation, if you like."

When the website Gawker put out a call for insider stories, an anonymous picker at an Amazon warehouse in Nevada called it the hardest job he had ever loved. "I lost weight, got into better shape than I have been in years and met some people out of my comfort zone," he wrote. "Ever wonder where people with mohawks, full-body tattoos and piercings work?" But that attitude was atypical. Most pickers complained about the byzantine hiring process, inadequate training, short breaks, forced overtime and false promises about bonuses and flexible schedules. "My initial thought was this is prison," wrote a worker from Tennessee. "I felt like asking anyone sitting by me or standing in line next to me, 'So, what are you in for?'"

In the blue-collar British town of Rugeley, north of Birmingham, an Amazon depot as large as nine soccer pitches sits on top of the abandoned tunnels and shafts of a coal mine that was once the heart of the local economy. Coal mining can be hellish, but it came with decent pay and a pension, as did most traditional assembly-line jobs. The average picker makes minimum wage. Many are employed by temp agencies and have to pound the concrete floor for months before being hired by Amazon proper. Their roles are transitory; in a sense, they are worth less than the machines that might one day replace them. Rugeley's pickers are thankful to have jobs, but they don't earn enough to stabilize the town's economy. Even the development officials who welcomed Amazon's arrival are questioning whether the warehouse will help the community in the long run. Not a very rosy vision of the new economy.

Christine Murray's depersonalized workday lasts around eight hours. It ends when she delivers her final letter and returns the van to the depot. Routes got longer when the transformation plan kicked in, and even if she skips her breaks, she is rarely finished early. ("Although 'cakewalks' are being eliminated, we have seen no equivalent drop in the number of particularly long or voluminous routes, also known as 'pigs' or 'widow-makers,'" wrote Bill Walker. "Route measurement, we are told, is necessarily an imperfect science.") Murray earns around $25 an hour, a grandfathered wage. On a good shift — for instance, the cool autumn day that I shadow her — she enjoys the job. Sometimes she even loves it. Despite beefs with management, all those sore muscles and a cloudy future, she is outside, getting exercise. A chance to see every nook and cranny on her turf.

We cut through a grassy utility corridor and pause for a wistful look at some frolicking dogs. Murray empties her satchel along a row of townhouses, loops back to the vehicle and drives to a subsidized apartment building for seniors. In the dingy mailroom, she pushes Canadian Tire and Swiss Chalet flyers into 252 mailboxes. Even rapid-fire, this takes 10 minutes. She's not sure what the time value is, only that most of this paper will go directly into the recycling bin in the lobby.

A man peeks through the tiny square door of a mailbox. "What are you doing in there?" he barks with theatrical impatience. "Hurry up. I might have a cheque for $50,000."

"Nope," Murray deadpans back. "Just flyers."

A few old-timers sit on a bench in the lobby, eager to shuffle over for a look. Pension cheques and disability payments are due.

Murray steps into the elevator to take a parcel to the 17th floor. We're joined by a white-haired man in a leather jacket. "Nice day," he rasps, holding two fingers against the bandage over the surgical hole in his throat.

"Here," Murray says to him, pulling a handful of blue elastic bands from her pocket, "I've got something for you."

"What do you use them for?" I ask.

"Well," he says, smiling, "I need something to wrap up all my money."

That exchange, though fleeting, came to mind when I heard about the end of home delivery. Murray was fulfilling her role as a uniformed community figure in the elevator, distributing more than the mail. We think we can automatize our way to prosperity and happiness, yet by eliminating her vocation, the human touch is left behind.

Murray is not nostalgic. Some of her colleagues at the sorting station talk about the good old days, "but that's the past," she says. "It happened back there, and it's gone. That's where it belongs. The most important thing is right now."

Other posties lament the values we are losing. "There is more to my job than sliding flyers through a slot," Melanie Mackenzie, a letter carrier in Halifax, Nova Scotia, wrote in that city's alternative newsweekly, the *Coast*, after Canada Post went public with its plan to end home delivery. "My job is to deliver you a better world."

This idea is expressed on a grand scale by the U.S. Postal Service, whose main building in Manhattan is adorned with an inscription of those famous words by Herodotus: "Neither snow nor rain nor heat nor gloom of night stays these couriers from the swift completion of their appointed rounds." And on a grander scale in Hollywood. In the Kevin Costner film *The Postman* — which won Golden Raspberry Awards for worst picture, worst actor and worst director in 1998 — a drifter finds the mail van of a dead letter carrier in post-apocalyptic America (supposedly 2013). Costner's character puts on the skeleton's uniform, picks up his satchel and begins the dangerous and heroic process of re-establishing communication between isolated settlements, one letter at a time. "There used to be a postman on every street in America," he says in one particularly rousing speech. "Getting a letter meant you were part of something bigger than yourself. I don't think we really understood what they meant to us until they were gone."

To parse what a lack of walking does to our economy, and the stability a greater emphasis on walking could provide, let's begin with the basics: our health. In the United States, walking levels fell 66 percent between 1960 and 2009, says a 2012 benchmarking report from the Washington, D.C.–based Alliance for Biking & Walking, produced with funding from the U.S. Centers for Disease Control and Prevention. This corresponded with a 156 percent jump in obesity rates. In 2009, 40 percent of all trips taken by Americans were shorter than two miles, yet 87 percent of trips between one and two miles were made by car, as were 62 percent of trips shorter than a mile. We might be able to manage some of these on foot.

Tasked by the Society of Actuaries with calculating the cost of obese and overweight citizens in the U.S. and Canada, actuarial researchers Donald Behan and Sam Cox came up with an estimated annual total of $300 billion — $127 billion for medical care, $49 billion from loss of productivity caused by excess mortality, $43 billion from loss of productivity caused by disability among active workers, $72 billion from loss of productivity caused by totally disabled workers. Patients with diabetes, they noted, account for one-third of all Medicare spending in the U.S.

Walking will not magically restore people to peak condition, but as Behan says with actuarial clarity, extra weight and obesity have "detrimental economic effects." He calls for employers and the insurance industry to help people "make smart, healthy decisions." To that end, when it released these findings, the Society of Actuaries also trumpeted a survey of American adults that found that 83 percent "would be willing to follow a healthy lifestyle, such as participating in a health and wellness program, if incentivized through their health plan." If just one in 10 began a regular walking program, the country would save $5.6 billion each year, enough to pay the tuition of more than a million college students.

The economy doesn't do anything without a healthy workforce, U.S. Surgeon General Boris Lushniak said at a forum in Washington in 2014. "Let's go retro, folks. We used to walk as a society. Does it take a $150 pair of running shoes, or a $60- to $90-a-month member-ship in a health club? It doesn't. It's walking! Think of it as a patriotic duty for the good of our nation."

Conceding that there is a paucity of definitive evidence, the Alliance for Biking & Walking report corrals together recent studies from throughout the U.S. to show that even without government support, communities that invest in walking and cycling projects save money not only through healthier citizens, but also through reduced traffic congestion and shorter commute times. They have higher property values, create new jobs and attract tourists. "As economic recession has hit almost every level of our society over the last few years, active transportation has emerged as a promising sector for growth and revitalization," the report says.

The majority of North Americans live in cities, where concrete is the backbone of transportation infrastructure. When the urban jungle expands or requires maintenance, engineers draw up plans, and the heavy-duty machines — and people to operate them — rumble in. To repair something as simple as a footpath, concrete sidewalks have to be dug up and replaced. The drainage system will likely require attention. Trees might be planted, ornamental brickwork laid, pedestrian ramps built, signage installed. Bike-lane projects have their own rhythm. Markings are painted on streets, curbs extended, bollards fabricated. Roadwork falls into two main categories: resurfacing streets, which entails excavation, paving and painting, and more elaborate projects, which also necessitate engin-eering, drainage and erosion control, and perhaps utility relocations. These descriptions give you a general picture of transportation infrastructure work in Baltimore, Maryland. Pretty standard stuff. But when an economist looked into how these types of projects impacted employment, her results were noteworthy.

Anybody behind the wheel of a bulldozer or rattling at the handle of a jackhammer on one of these jobs is directly employed as a result of the work. Supply-chain industries, such as cement manu-facturing and trucking, are the beneficiaries of indirect employment.

Then there are the induced jobs, in nearby restaurants and stores, for instance, as construction workers spend their pay. Everything from the cafés where hardhats line up for their Americanos to the dairies that supply the cream can be counted. The City of Baltimore gave data on a range of its transportation projects to Heidi Garrett-Peltier of the Political Economy Research Institute at the University of Massachusetts. She determined that every $1 million spent on creating on-street bike lanes led to 14.4 jobs, compared to 11.3 jobs for every $1 million spent on pedestrian projects and seven jobs for every $1 million spent on road infrastructure. The difference, she explained, is because bike and pedestrian work tends to be more labour- and design-intensive than road repair. That is, the ratios of labour costs to material costs, and engineering costs to construction costs, are higher.

Apportioning more spending into bike and pedestrian projects will to some degree undercut the auto sector and its spinoffs, but as we'll see later in this chapter, most of the money spent on cars and gasoline leaves the local market. And just as a shift from fossil fuels toward renewable energy will lead to a bumpy labour market, a localized green economy — and the jobs it creates — is our best long-term shot at sustainability. (Chris Turner's book *The Leap* offers an excellent account of this transition, which is well underway in Germany, where 31 percent of the country's electricity was generated from renewable energy sources in the first half of 2014.)

Garrett-Peltier validated her Baltimore statistics with a national study on the employment impacts of bicycling, pedestrian and road infrastructure. Examining 58 construction projects in 11 American cities, a cross-section that included Anchorage, Houston and Madison, Wisconsin, she found that cycling projects create an average of 11.4 jobs for every $1 million of spending, versus 10 jobs for pedestrian projects and 7.8 jobs for roadwork. "The U.S. is currently experiencing high unemployment, unsustainable use of carbon-based energy, and a national obesity epidemic," she writes. "All three of these problems can be partly addressed through increased walking and cycling."

Providing infrastructure for active transit, argues Garrett-Peltier, is more than a health proposition.

The bottom-line returns of walkability in Baltimore go way beyond employment. In 2010, its city council adopted a "Complete Streets" policy, a commitment to address the needs of transit users, cyclists and walkers of every age and ability alongside drivers in all future transportation development. More than 600 American jurisdictions have signed Complete Streets charters. Part of the motivation is the health and safety of residents, as well as environmental stewardship. But a walkable community also raises property values, points out a 2011 report from the Downtown Baltimore Family Alliance.

Walk Score, a Seattle-based company that ranks neighbourhood walkability based on inputs such as proximity to parks, schools, transit routes and grocery stores, has become a useful tool for realtors. Its scale ranges from zero to 100; communities below 24 are deemed car-dependent, while those above 90 earn the title Walker's Paradise. In 2009, economist Joe Cortright analyzed 94,000 real-estate transactions in 15 American housing markets and found that a one-point Walk Score increase will boost housing values by $700 to $3,000, depending on the market. Going from an average to above-average Walk Score will increase a home's value by $4,000 to $34,000. Las Vegas was the only city with a negative correlation between housing prices and walkability. Cortright, who did the research for a network of business, education and government executives called CEOs for Cities, offers some advice: "The nation's urban leaders should pay close attention to walkability as a key measure of urban vitality and as impetus for public policy that will increase overall property values — a key source of individual wealth and of revenues for cash-strapped governments in a tough economy."

Cortright compiled his data in the wake of the 2008 stock market collapse. The United States was deep in recession, and housing values were plummeting. It may seem counterintuitive to view higher real-estate prices as an indicator of urban livability, but not if you consider that the cost of a house reflects the quality of its neighbourhood as much as the condition of the physical structure itself. Also, that low and declining values are a sign of a troubled community, in extreme cases leading to social and economic collapse, such as Detroit's depopulation and bankruptcy. The acute fiscal anxiety of 2008 and 2009 may have passed for now, but the recession gave millions of Americans an opportunity to contemplate the role that walkability could play in a new approach to their cities: chiefly, the value of better transit, more mixing between commercial and residential land uses, and connected, complete streets. The next financial shock may give us another push in this direction.

"The upheaval in financing markets, the dramatic decline in housing prices, retrenchment in the retail sector and the ongoing restructuring of the automobile industry are all harbingers of change for the nation's cities," writes Cortright. "Continued uncertainty about future energy prices and the need to deal aggressively with climate change will demand new strategies in the years ahead. Our research suggests that walkability is already an important component of the value proposition of the nation's cities, and that improving walkability can be an important key to their future as well."

In addition to the real-estate gains, the Downtown Baltimore Family Alliance found that pedestrian zones in the city centre increased foot traffic from 20 to 40 percent and, as a result, retail sales grew between 10 and 25 percent. Customers on foot spend more than people who drive or take transit, reported a study of consumer spending in British towns: £91 each week, versus £64 among drivers and £46 for train passengers. Some of these shoppers are locals, but walkable downtowns also draw travellers, another source of revenue for cities. Plus, as businesses get stronger, the city earns more property-tax revenue.

If you believe in the Tao of urban studies theorist Richard Florida, who gained a global following by arguing that the fate of cities is linked to their ability to entice members of the so-called creative class, there is yet another payoff. Six in 10 Americans say they would choose to live in a walkable neighbourhood, either central or in the suburbs, if they could. Florida, head of the Martin Prosperity Institute at the University of Toronto's Rotman School of Management, notes that walkable metro areas have above-average levels of highly educated people, higher incomes and more high-tech companies. "Walkability is more than an attractive amenity," he writes. "It's a magnet for attracting and retaining the highly innovative businesses and highly skilled people that drive economic growth."

The city an hour down the highway from Baltimore holds some lessons too. In "Walk This Way: The Economic Promise of Walkable Places in Metropolitan Washington, D.C.," Brookings Institution economist Christopher Leinberger and Mariela Alfonzo, a research fellow at New York University's Polytechnic School of Engineering, argue that the 2008 drop in housing prices was not only the result of a high-risk, low-interest loan bubble bursting, but also the start of a "structural real estate market shift." The biggest decreases were in distant suburbs; homes in central neighbourhoods held steady and, in some cases, increased in value. They attribute this to an emerging preference for "mixed-use, compact, amenity-rich, transit-accessible neighborhoods or walkable places. . . . The trend is swinging away from neighborhoods that contain primarily large-lot single-family housing, few sidewalks, ample parking, and where driving is the primary means of transportation." Walkability is now a factor in two-thirds of home-purchasing decisions in the U.S.

This is leading the country to a predicament. Call it the residential cliff. There is an undersupply of small-lot and attached housing — a shortfall estimated at 12 to 13.5 million units — and a glut of about 28 million surplus large-lot homes. Builders have been slow to meet this new demand, in part because of the public- and private-sector barriers that complicate walkable development. Municipal policies, zoning ordinances and funding biases are blocking their path. High-density, mixed-use developments can be messy; banks and investors aren't comfortable with the risk or the capital demands. Leinberger and Alfonzo consider walkability a mechanism that can boost a neighbourhood's triple bottom line: profit, people and planet. Yet the real-estate finance industry, they write, "lacks the experience, institutional mission or even fiduciary latitude to appropriately consider walkable development investments or loans."

The D.C. analysis makes several strong recommendations. Rewrite the zoning codes that are costly and time-consuming to overturn for builders who want to make walkable, mixed-use developments. Seek out and support neighbourhoods that are positioned to become more walkable; since the land mass will be small, the infrastructure costs will be minimal. Implement subsidized housing programs to compensate for the lack of walkable developments until the supply-demand mismatch can be alleviated and prices drop to more affordable levels. Bring private developers, investors, social equity advocates, the public sector and citizen-led groups into this conversation. "Considering the economic benefits," write Leinberger and Alfonzo, "walkability should be a critical part of all strategic growth plans."

North Americans drive roughly 50 times as many miles as they walk, says Todd Litman, executive director of the Victoria Transport Policy Institute, in British Columbia. This is why the car has traditionally been at the centre of our transportation policies, he writes in a paper about the economic value of walkability. By putting the car on a pedestal, city planners undervalue non-motorized travel. They overlook the fact that non-drivers (and those who drive minimally) subsidize people who don't think twice before getting behind the wheel. Regardless of how many miles you drive, the same percentage of your taxes goes toward road maintenance. Moreover, studies on traffic economics tend to concentrate on the length of a trip, ignoring factors such as the costs of vehicle ownership, road congestion and parking, as well as the health implications of motorized travel. Walking is often disregarded because it is seen as a lower-status activity. Because it is not championed by a powerful lobby group. Because it is easy to take for granted. You don't even need a sidewalk to walk beside a road. The act can be ignored because of its universality. This is one of the reasons the Society of Actuaries wants exercise programs incentivized through health plans. Even though walking is free and easy, there is a perceived barrier. It's hard to compete against sexy car commercials.

The personal cost savings from reduced vehicle use, however, are not easily dismissed. American households in car-dependent communities spend 50 percent more on transportation (about $8,500 a year) than those in more walkable neighbourhoods (less than $5,500 a year). The difference stems from fuel consumption, insurance, parking fees, car depreciation and other factors. Auto-dependent communities also use land less efficiently. Walkable residential and commercial developments require less space, less parking and smaller setbacks from the road to mitigate traffic noise and danger.

Litman's spreadsheets, based on data from the U.S. Department of Transportation, peg federal, state and local government annual spending on roadways at $30.8 billion, $66.4 billion and $31.3 billion respectively, with an average of 3.5 percent of that funding — 0.6, 1 and 10 percent across the three levels — devoted to walking. And that's without factoring in public expenditures on parking facilities and traffic enforcement. Bump government support for walking infrastructure up to 10 to 20 percent of total transportation resources, Litman writes, and the change in planning priorities will have a profound impact on the economic well-being of the nation. Sidewalks will teem with healthier, relaxed people with money in their pockets.

The Alliance for Biking & Walking report brings geopolitics into this discussion. The average American family spends 16 cents of every dollar on transportation, its second-biggest expense after shelter. When you consider the sources of the vehicles and gas they purchase, most of those dollars go to "foreign car companies, and to pay for foreign fuel." Beyond energy-dependency concerns, there's a simple reason to take notice of this flow: those dollars leave the neighbourhood.

Using data from the Internal Revenue Service, Joe Cortright looked at spending on gas and cars in the U.S. in 2010 and calculated that 73 and 86 percent of the spending, respectively, immediately left the local economy. Because New Yorkers rely on transit and walking more than residents of most American cities, the roughly $19 billion below average they spend on car travel translates into $16 billion "available to be spent in the local economy. Because this money tends to be re-spent in other sectors, it stimulates business."

Christopher Leinberger also puts walking on a ledger. He highlights the disposable incomes of walkability-craving millennials and baby boomers (significant savings, no children to support) as a key to revitalizing the urban cores of America. As he writes in *The Option of Urbanism: Investing in a New American Dream*, 100 million new households will form in the U.S. by 2025, and 88 percent will be childless. That's a lot of spending money, and much of it is headed downtown. "The metropolitan area that does not offer walkable urbanism," he says, "is probably destined to lose economic development opportunities."

Portland, Oregon, where Cortright is based, is an urbanist poster child. The city of 590,000, with a metropolitan population of nearly 3 million, is known for its progressive politics, its 60 or so microbreweries and, despite the Pacific Northwest rain, an outdoor lifestyle. In some ways, Portland is a normal American city: its urban density is average, and traditional industries such as steel manufacturing and shipping play a significant role in the economy. But in addition to a strong public transit network, 8 percent of commuters bike to work, the highest percentage in the U.S., and Walk Score ranks it the 12th most walkable community on a list of the country's 50 largest cities.

Portland has this transportation profile largely because of a pair of foresighted decisions. With support from the state, the city was an early adopter of the "skinny streets" philosophy, a movement calling for a reduction of roadway width requirements in municipal standards. Narrow streets reduce "speeding, vehicle crashes, street construction costs, pedestrian crossing distances, impervious surfaces (and therefore stormwater drain capacity), street maintenance and resurfacing costs, and heat re-radiation, which contributes to the urban heat island effect." Our streets got fat not only to accommodate all the cars on the road, but also as a vestige of antiquated safety controls: so horse-drawn wagons could make U-turns, so fire engines could pass one another, despite better building materials and sprinkler systems minimizing the frequency with which these situations occur. Going on a road diet helps a city reap the benefits of increased pedestrianism.

Since 1980, Portland has also adhered to an urban growth boundary. This did not prevent sprawl. The boundary is porous. It has been expanded three dozen times, with thousands of acres added for housing and industrial land use. Still, it has limited the type of sprawl I frequently tromped though in Calgary and Edmonton. Which, as Cortright details in a white paper for CEOs for Cities called "Portland's Green Dividend," led to the number of miles driven per person peaking in 1996, with locals now driving 20 percent less than the average American. Vehicle miles — total miles driven divided by population — continue to increase as a whole in the U.S. The four-mile daily difference between Portlanders and other Americans, when coupled with rush-hour travel times falling by a dozen minutes each day, saves residents approximately $2.5 billion every year in vehicle costs and lost productivity. And much of that money, as in New York, stays in the city.

Portland's atmosphere attracts young people. In the 1990s, the city's population of 25- to 34-year-olds with a college education grew 50 percent, five times more than the national average. This is Richard Florida's creative class, and it flocked to the city's walkable, central neighbourhoods. In contrast to "white flight" to the suburbs 50 years ago, demographer William Frey calls this in-migration "bright flight." Flourishing around this workforce, chicken-and-egg debate notwithstanding, there are now 1,200-plus tech companies in Portland. And 30 percent of all jobs in the city are within three miles of the central business district, placing Portland behind only

New York and San Francisco in this category among the country's 50 largest metro areas.

In the Greater Toronto Area, where traffic gridlock drains an estimated $6 billion out of the economy every year in travel delays and vehicle costs, the city's chief planner has made walking the hub of her strategy to ease congestion. Historically, says Jennifer Keesmaat, a lot of planning decisions have been made by men who like big-vision, billion-dollar schemes. Subways! Freeways! The reality is that something as subtle as getting more children to walk to school will have a bigger impact on traffic. More than 20 percent of all morning rush-hour trips in Toronto involve parents driving their kids to school. "We need to rebuild a culture around walking," Keesmaat says. "It's a much more profound infrastructure investment than any roads or subway we can build."

After dashing around the U.K. by train in the summer of 2013, I caught my breath with a hike along the rocky coastline of a remote peninsula in northern Wales. Walking is hardwired into British culture, like hockey in Canada: rare is the time and place it cannot be done, observed or discussed. I know a guy who was born and raised in the fabled Green and Pleasant Land. Until he was old enough to tag along, his parents had a standing date with a babysitter every weekend so they could go rambling in the hills and dales. This was serious business.

In Wales, walking has a particularly high purpose. It puts food on the table. Domestic travellers and international visitors made more than 28 million walking trips to the countryside and coastlines of Wales in 2009, according to a study by the Welsh Economy Research Unit at Cardiff University. Those walkers spent £632 million and were responsible for another £275 million of indirect economic activity. They kept 11,980 people gainfully employed in the tourist trade, as well as sectors as diverse as manufacturing and financial services, big numbers in a nation with just over 3 million people.

My five-day hike spanned a short section of the Wales Coast

Path, an 870-mile trail that traces the country's entire shoreline, making Wales the only country in the world with a footpath showcasing all of its seafront terrain. About 2.9 million people walked on the WCP between October 2011 and September 2012, spending £33.2 million on gear, accommodation, food, drinks and other amenities. On the Llŷn Peninsula, where I went, these expenditures help to keep farmers, fishers, grocery stores, bakeries, inns and pubs in business.

The WCP was completed in 2012 by blazing new trails, linking existing legs and installing signage. A £14.6 million construction push finished the project, and it will be supported by roughly £2 million per year in maintenance and promotional spending. These investments are not a hard sell for the Welsh government, which pegs the value of the goods and services generated by its natural environment at around £9 billion per year. Walking is seen as a key bridge between conservation and revenue. "While it is very difficult to associate monetary values to biodiversity and landscape," the Cardiff University study concludes, "it has been possible here to assign monetary value to one set of leisure activities closely linked to the quality of regional environmental assets."

In heavily populated and developed parts of the U.K., there is a much more contentious tug-of-war between environment and economy. To get perspective on this debate, I hiked to the top of a wee Scottish mountain with Joseph Murphy.

Murphy is the geographer who lives south of Glasgow, near the Ken Bridge Hotel, in the village of New Galloway. Born in England but of Irish descent, he trekked 930 miles up the west coasts of Ireland and Scotland in 2006, exploring his Gaelic roots. Along the way, the University of Glasgow environmental studies professor investigated the challenges and opportunities of sustainable development. Was community, he wondered, the starting point?

Murphy took me to the Merrick, the highest hill in southern Scotland. With his border collie Jed bounding ahead, we set out from the parking lot at Glentrool, a pretty green valley in Galloway Forest Park. Three hundred square miles of heather-clad hills and granite outcrops, home to red deer and golden eagles, this is the largest forest park in Britain. It's also part of a UNESCO biosphere reserve, the first "new style" biosphere in Scotland, established to promote wilderness preservation, scientific research and sustainable development. The trail began beside a rushing brook, climbing through a carpet of ferny bracken, dwarf willow and juniper. Within a few minutes, we were in a forest of spindly Sitka spruce. The trees, planted a couple decades ago, would soon be cut.

The harvesting is largely mechanical and creates few jobs. But the majority of the timber is processed in local sawmills, with haulage and processing employing more than 500 people (nearly as many permanent jobs as the total touted by the proposed Northern Gateway pipeline in Canada). The Scottish Forestry Commission manages the logging and says conservation and tourism are given due consideration. This is not window dressing. The 850,000 people who visit Galloway Forest Park each year contribute nearly £16 million to the area's businesses, propelling tourism to third place in the regional economy after forestry and agriculture.

As we rose above the spruce, a panorama of green hills and blue lochs opened up, and Murphy told me about walking the length of Ireland and Scotland. In Rossport, a village in Ireland's County Mayo, he met a group of protestors camping outside the gates of a Shell natural-gas refinery that was under construction. A year earlier, five of them had spent 94 days in jail for blocking access to their land to prevent work on a high-pressure pipeline. Murphy sympathized with the protestors. "Poorly conceived development projects have been imposed on rural communities around the world for decades," he writes in his book about the walk, *At the Edge*, "and at last we are learning to ask a simple but powerful question. Is the community doing development for itself or is development being done to it?" Ireland's energy policy, he believes, is outdated: "Predict future energy demand and provide for it through large-scale projects." Nowhere on his walk did he see any evidence of attempts to reduce energy consumption: thousands of new suburban homes and not a single micro-wind turbine, solar water heater or photovoltaic cell.

Four hundred miles north of Rossport, on Lewis, the largest island in Scotland's Outer Hebrides, he encountered a similar resistance campaign. Only there, crofters were fighting against the construction of a massive wind farm. A consortium of multinational energy and engineering companies wanted to erect 234 turbines on the moorland where locals cut peat not for export but to heat their homes, a harvest they have capably managed for centuries. In the face of cultural as well as ecological concerns — locals complained about the industrialization of their landscape, and the installation's impact on rare and endangered birds — the wind-farm proposal was scaled down in size. Still, the £500 million project, which would have supplied 10 percent of Scotland's electricity, was rejected by the government over concerns about its impact on a globally significant peatland.

Today, a new small-scale wind farm on the Isle of Lewis is seeking financing. There will be three turbines, owned by the community. The electricity will be sold to the national grid, and the revenue will support local development. "This project is about power, but not just electricity," said the chair of the development trust helming the proposal. He calls it a "quiet revolution."

The economy is a wholly owned subsidiary of the environment. So said Gaylord Nelson, the former Governor of Wisconsin and Democrat senator who organized the first Earth Day in 1970. "All economic activity is dependent upon that environment and its underlying resource base of forests, water, air, soil, and minerals," he wrote. "When the environment is finally forced to file for bankruptcy because its resource base has been polluted, degraded, dissipated, and irretrievably compromised, the economy goes into bankruptcy with it."

Twenty-eight percent of greenhouse-gas emissions in the U.S. come from transportation. Passenger cars and light-duty trucks account for more than half of the sector's total. Only electricity generation burns more carbon, one-third of the national output, 80 percent from coal. There are threads to tease out — cars emit more exhaust when their engines are cold, magnifying the value of making short journeys on foot — but no need to dwell in these pages on the environmental virtues of consuming less energy and polluting less by travelling under our own steam. It's an easy way to start to make a difference. And conceptually, walking can help elucidate the symbiotic relationship between environment and economy. Especially if one encounters a series of intertwined issues on a single journey.

Contemplating the gas-refinery and wind-farm conflicts as he slowly advanced north, Murphy came to see that in the 21st century, colonialism and imperialism can be defined as the projection of power across space, such as when the periphery is exploited for the benefit of the core. Remote communities are invited to join the fight against climate change by building very large wind farms, even though the energy and profit generated is typically piped far from its source. Even though we don't seem to be serious about reducing energy demands. This, Murphy told me, can be considered colonization of the future: "Our current generation is imperilling the ability of future generations to live reasonable, comfortable, acceptable lives. We are exploiting the future as a periphery."

But when you walk from core to periphery, you link the two places in a comprehensible way. You see problems — and opportunities — at a human scale. You see the impact of government and corporate decisions that are made hundreds of miles away. You see the historical evolution of a region and get a glimpse of what its future might hold.

Murphy and I reached a narrow ridge and followed a stone wall to top of the Merrick. The Irish Sea's North Channel was a hazy blue line to the west. Murphy had never been to the peak before. He scanned the horizon and spotted a few turbines here and there. "Well, that's nice," he said. "We're not ringed by wind farms."

Puzzling over Murphy's words in my home office months later, the lucidity of the mountaintop was hard to conjure. Not only because of the prescription-pad illegibility of my shorthand. Our brains, remember, work differently when we are on foot — a phenomenon that has not gone unnoticed in the business world.

Walking three and a half miles around his New England neighbourhood every morning helps the president of Advertising for Humanity, Dan Pallotta, rehearse speeches and come up with new concepts. "The first mile of my walk is just a racket of competing voices of judgment and to-do lists," he wrote in one of his regular blog posts for the *Harvard Business Review*. "But after about two miles, no matter how low my mood may have been at the outset, those voices settle down." Apple chief executive officer Steve Jobs had his most serious conversations while walking. Louis W. Sullivan, U.S. Secretary of Health in the early 1990s, went for walks with colleagues while visiting his agency's regional offices. He learned about policy debates and morale within the department, and staff got to meet the boss, something many had never experienced during their long careers.

Jobs and Sullivan practiced a habit known as MBWA: management by walking around. It was first popularized in the 1950s by Bill Hewlett and Dave Packard, founders of the eponymous electronics company, and became a buzzword in the 1980s after the publication of the block-buster business book *In Search of Excellence*, whose authors called MBWA the "technology of the obvious." With email replacing face-to-face contact in many offices, casual desk-side conversations can help managers connect with employees, and encourage staff to become more engaged. As long as the walkabouts are regular, and not an attempt to surprise or snoop, they can help foster a more cohesive and communicative organization. "If you wait for people to come to you, you'll only get small problems," said American management consultant W. Edwards Deming. "The big problems are [revealed when] people don't realize they have one in the first place."

The walking meeting, a natural fit within our free-flowing mobile business culture, goes further. A few years ago, when Silicon Valley executive and entrepreneur Nilofer Merchant had to discuss something with a busy colleague, the other woman suggested they talk shop while walking her dogs. It was a revelation. "You can take care of your health, or you can take care of your obligations," Merchant says about time-crunched corporate culture in a TED Talk, "and one always comes at the cost of the other." The average North American sits for 9.3 hours each day, and it's killing us. Merchant now covers 20 to 30 miles in walking meetings most weeks.

As with beat cops in North Philly, these sessions produce ancillary benefits. The moderate activity gives you energy, and the fresh air and natural light can stimulate more creativity and open dialogue than the fluorescent *je ne sais quoi* of a shut-in conference room. "Getting out of the box," says Merchant, "leads to out-of-the-box thinking." By realizing she did not have to choose between her fitness and her professional life, she has come to understand that business problems don't have to be seen as a battle between opposing choices. What's more, incorporating exercise into your nine-to-five is a way to integrate physical health into your everyday life and stop treating it as a separate activity that gets dropped when your schedule becomes too crowded. You see your life as a continuum, not a scattering of chores to complete.

Instead of lecturing about wellness inside a classroom, University of Toronto health communication specialist Margaret MacNeill, who had cautioned me about the medicalization of exercise, takes student doctors and nurses outside to walk and talk. Hierarchical barriers fall and ideas flow. "It's a wonderful icebreaker," she says. "Your metabolism revs up and sparks your brain cells." Small groups, quiet routes, comfortable shoes and a subject that requires minimal note-taking (such as the start of a project) are the keys to an effective session. Leaving your smartphone behind helps too.

Daniel Kahneman isn't convinced. The Israeli-American psychologist, who won the Nobel Prize in economics in 2002, believes that while it is pleasant to walk and think at the same time, these activities compete for resources from the part of the mind that guides our deliberate and logical decisions. "If I must construct an intricate argument under time pressure," he writes in his book *Thinking, Fast and Slow*, "I would rather be still, and I would prefer sitting to standing." When accelerating above strolling speed, his ability to draw conclusions is impaired. "A mental effort of self-control is needed to resist the urge to slow down. Self-control and deliberate thought apparently draw on the same limited budget."

Most of us adhere to Kahneman's belief. When we get busy, we hunker down at our desks. This is a high-risk practice, considering the long-term health impacts of so much sitting. Yet we are creatures of habit.

My schedule got tight when I stopped travelling and reporting, and began to actually write this book. Juggling magazine assignments and domestic duties, I had little time to walk. I sat and sat, and reverted to frequent, short runs along Ottawa's Rideau River to relieve creative and parenting pressures. (The knee surgery had worked, though I remain skittish about folk-music festivals.) Then I got a mysterious skin infection, possibly caused by an insect bite, that made my right hand swell like a steak. Doctors gave me intravenous antibiotics in the emergency room over three days and sent me home with an ambulatory infusion pump, which shot drugs into my arm every eight hours. A tangle of plastic tubing was affixed to my hip in a fanny pack. I could not run. So I tried a treadmill desk.

The concept is simple: a tall desk, a flat treadmill. An American company called LifeSpan loaned me one of its sleek, grey TRI200-DT5 models. It has a sturdy, adjustable-height tabletop and a speed range of 0.4 to 4 miles per hour, so users can comfortably type or talk, the thinking goes, without risking sitting disease. DIY units such as the archetype built by Mayo Clinic obesity researcher James Levine in the 1990s have evolved into today's calorie-counting, Bluetooth-equipped commercial models, with prices in the $1,000 to $5,000 ballpark. Treadmill motors are designed to work optimally at slow speeds for long hours. But I wondered, settling into my ad hoc basement workstation and setting a clip of 1.5 miles an hour, would I actually get anything done?

Like most freelancers, I started my day with email correspondence, Twitter and other vital online business (such as renewing my driver's licence). After 45 minutes on the machine, I forgot that I was walking. My lower back and feet hurt, so I raised the desktop and swapped my slippers for a pair of running shoes.

Two hours later, the pain was gone. Sweating slightly, I attempted to remove my hoodie while in motion. Bad idea. The safety key clipped to my pants stopped the belt before I tumbled into the wood panelling. I managed to write a few hundred words, but swayed drunkenly when I stepped off for lunch, as if disembarking onto the dock after a boat ride.

A couple of early afternoon phone interviews went well. Conversation was no problem at that pace, though my longhand notes were worse than usual. By the time I powered down, I had covered 8.8 miles and burned off 716 calories. A productive first day.

"Chairdom is hugely affecting humans," Levine said to Susan Orlean of the *New Yorker*, both on their treadmill desks while talking. "No one has really understood what we have lost by sitting all the time."

Although Levine and Orleans are tread-desk converts, research on the effectiveness of working while on a treadmill leans toward Kahneman's stance. University of Tennessee exercise physiologist David R. Bassett had graduate students do a range of office tasks while seated and while walking one mile per hour on a treadmill. Not only did subjects drag and drop with a mouse faster and type more quickly when seated, they also had "meaningfully" better math scores. Their ability to pay attention and reading comprehension scores did not change when they were tested while walking.

I kept the treadmill desk for a couple months, experimenting with various speeds and alternating between the basement and my office chair on the main floor. Maybe it was the natural light or fresher air, but I worked better while sitting. *Cosmopolitan* editor-in-chief Joanna Coles reads at and loves her treadmill desk, but she also has plenty of space for an old-fashioned desk in her corner office on the 42nd floor of the Hearst Tower in midtown Manhattan. For me, productivity upstairs earned more time outside. On the machine, I felt the cognitive bottlenecks described by Kahneman. Besides, is it really walking if you don't go anywhere? Treadmills, a friend grumbled, are hamster wheels for humans.

After I shipped the unit back to LifeSpan, Ottawa's coldest winter in 20 years settled in. Stocking up on long underwear and embracing the snow and ice, I had learned in Alberta, is the best way to stay warm and stave off seasonal gloom. I found myself looking for excuses to get outdoors. A quick online search netted somebody who could help.

Andrew Markle, a tall, slim man in his early 30s, meets me outside a café on a busy corner. He opens the rear door of his plastic-interiored Honda Element. There is a basset hound slobbering in the front passenger seat. Spence has to ride shotgun, Markle explains, otherwise he will pee.

Markle and his wife, Brecken Hancock, own a dog-walking company called Walk It Off. She is a poet and he writes science fiction. She also does policy work for the federal government. They wanted to start a business when they moved to the city in 2012. A year after launching, they had a waiting list. At $19 per walk for a five-days-a-week package, Markle earns as much as Hancock would if she kept his hours.

I sit down in the car and meet the rest of my fellow passengers: Zermatt, a red retriever; Finn and Pixie, goldendoodles; Franklin, a bull mastiff; and Fanny, the smallest, part beagle, confined to a travel carrier because she always wants to wrestle. Ollie, Markle tells me, driving toward his secret forest in the suburbs, is on vacation.

My friends get restless when we curl off the highway. Markle stops on the wide shoulder of a rural road. He clips all six dogs to leashes, which are attached to a heavy-duty carabineer on his belt. We walk along a snowy path into a thicket of leafless oak and maple. After a minute, he lets the dogs run free. They romp in the snow: running, jumping, barking, digging. This is no fenced-in, inner-city doggie compound. It is a restorative place. I picture a class of schoolchildren bursting through the doors for recess — or a group of office workers set free from their cubicles.

The dogs do their business and Markle bags it. Fanny and Franklin play tug-of-war with a branch, growling. We do a two-mile loop, about average for an outing. The trees and a series of ridges block the wind. Spence needs a treat to be convinced to stay with the pack. "C'mon, buddy," says Markle, "hustle." Back in the car after an hour, Spence rests his neck on the gearshift and falls asleep.

Since starting Walk It Off, Markle has been driving more than ever. But he listens to audiobooks while on the road, and travels in that smooth window between morning and afternoon rush hours. His clients, nine-to-fivers mostly, don't have the freedom to spend an hour in the woods with their canine friends in the middle of the day. We can't all have jobs like Markle. We can't all afford to work part-time. But there is a movement afoot to inculcate the four-day workweek. More time to take care of ourselves and our families; more jobs for other people. So, what's wrong with a four-hour workday? Markle savours the balance he has: freedom, exercise, decent remuneration, creative satisfaction on the side. While he's not exactly opting out of the rat race, he hasn't jumped in, either.

"What's your favourite thing about this type of job?" I ask just before he drops me off.

"It pays well and it's only a half day, so I can also work on other things that I'm interested in," he says. "And yeah, the walking. That's probably the best part."

five

POLITICS

"Is a democracy, such as we know it, the last improvement possible in government? Is it not possible to take a step further towards recognizing and organizing the rights of man?"

— *Henry David Thoreau, "Civil Disobedience"*

"I learnt how distant my colleagues and I in government were from the lives of others. Our policy papers existed in a grotesque jargon space of misleading phrases about 'transparent, predictable and accountable financial processes.' I had become more confident disagreeing . . . because my walk had showed me real people in real places."

— *Rory Stewart, Member of Parliament, U.K.*

"Female salmon fake their orgasms."

Six men are standing on the rocky flats beside the River Lune, in northwestern England, discussing the threats confronting the local fishery. This used to be one of the best sea trout rivers in the United Kingdom. Not anymore. Nitrates and phosphates from the fertilizing slurry spread over adjacent fields leach into the water. Heavy rainstorms, increasingly frequent of late, disturb the streambed gravel and destroy spawning nests. A proposed hydroelectric project could disrupt the flow. And at the mouth of the Lune, some 15 miles away, salmon-farm escapees migrate through the Kent Channel, bringing sea lice and possibly other diseases.

Well, they *were* talking about fishing. Now the conversation has screeched to a halt.

"Female salmon fake their orgasms," repeats the man in the green golf shirt, a pair of binoculars hanging from his neck. John Hatt was once a travel writer. Then he launched a profitable website, Cheapflights. Patron of the Lune Rivers Trust, he is a distinguished, respected citizen. And, apparently, not shy about speaking his mind.

"It's true," says Hatt, and he begins to explain. When she is ready to spawn, the female fish digs a hole in the gravel river bottom. She hovers over the pit, opens her mouth and starts to quiver intensely. A mate joins her and does the same thing. She releases eggs, he releases sperm, and thousands of fry live subaqueously ever after. Unless the male is not positioned directly over the eggs. That's when she fakes it.

"They don't make a noise, do they?" asks one of the men, fighting back laughter.

The others chortle. Everybody except the wiry fellow wearing a crisp grey suit, a blue dress shirt with white pinstripes and a tightly knotted blue tie decorated with anchors, sailboats and tiny tropical islands with perfect little palm trees. His tousled mop of a-little-too-long brown hair and scuffed brown dress shoes are the only hints that he might not be uncomfortable here. Arms crossed, he is looking at the shallow water riffling over smooth rocks. Bees and butterflies flit among the purple thistle and goldenrod that line the grassy embankment. Finally, he speaks.

"You're acting like a politician now, John," he jabs. "You're just trying to change the subject."

Everybody laughs. Not that these anglers were a difficult group to relate to for rookie Member of Parliament Rory Stewart. He represents Penrith and the Border, the largest and most sparsely populated constituency in England, about 2,000 square miles of fields, fells, clear streams and stone walls. A place where "Glen Beck" invokes an image of a creek running through a deep, narrow valley, not the incendiary Fox network talk-show host. Politics are more courteous here. Plus, this has been a safe Conservative seat for the past century, a district once governed by Pitt the Younger, and even though Rory the Tory is a Scotsman, with blue blood, he knows how to meet people on their terms, on their turf.

The minute he arrived at Old Tebay Bridge, Stewart thanked the men for joining him on the stretch of water they wanted to discuss, rather than in a stuffy boardroom. "Can we go see the river?" he asked, then swiftly climbed a wooden stile over a barbed-wire fence and stepped down to the shore.

Stewart and I drove to the Lune from Brougham Hall Farm, 20 miles to the north, where he had spent the bulk of the day mingling with constituents at the Penrith Show, an agricultural fair that celebrated its 170th anniversary in 2013. When I reached the sprawling estate, a half-hour walk from my hotel on the High Street in the lively market town of Penrith, and tore myself away from watching motorcycle trickster Valentino jump over fire in the main ring, I found Stewart on a folding chair inside the Conservative Party tent, listening to a group of farmers, all in their early 20s, describe their daily frustrations.

"We're paid a ridiculous amount of money to fence off fields and keep sheep out," said one, "to protect wild orchids." A national public body called Natural England came up with this plan to conserve the endangered flower. Problem is, wild orchids *need* sheep. They nibble the brambles and hawthorn scrub that would otherwise choke out the flowers. It's one of countless disconnects between policy and the people. Stewart promised to try to do something about it.

"It's good that the local MP wants to listen," Matthew Blair, one of the young farmers, told me when their hour in the tent was finished. "He comes out of Westminster and spends time with people like us."

Blair's family met Stewart during the 2010 election campaign, when he called in on their farm. Even in rural ridings, door-knocking is a crucial canvassing strategy. But Stewart's arrival at the Blair homestead was unusual. He got there entirely on foot.

After he was selected as the Conservative nominee for Penrith and the Border, a process that culminated in each shortlisted contender speaking to the public for five minutes from the show ring of the livestock auction mart, where Stewart says "the expressions of the farmers implied they had seen mule shearlings who would make better candidates," he wanted to *really* get to know the area. So he went on a 300-mile trek through the constituency, distributing pamphlets on country lanes, stopping at community meetings, joining trivia competitions in village pubs and sleeping wherever he was offered lodging for the night: a medieval keep, a 17th-century farmhouse, a room above the pub (where his lack of pop music and soap opera knowledge cemented a last-place finish in the trivia contest). Some of the tour was carefully coordinated. One evening, he zipped back to Penrith for dinner with then–New York City mayor Michael Bloomberg. But most of Stewart's encounters on the campaign trail were spontaneous, like his walkabout at Brougham Hall Farm.

After posing for a group photo with the next-gen farmers, he strode about the fairgrounds, calling in at the Cumbria Dog Training and Cumbria Wildlife Trust booths, and dropping £1 on a raffle ticket for a Peugeot at the Eden Valley Hospice tent. He shook hands with tractor dealers and auctioneers, and inspected pens with 20 different breeds of sheep, introducing me to their owner, who attempted to teach me how to recognize their subtle differences. (It was all sheep to me, though I did learn that peak-capped Hugh Harrison was born on his ancestral farmland, and that he helped out on the film *Withnail and I*, a cult classic that was shot south of Penrith: "I enjoyed it, but it takes a bit of the fun out of the sausage when you see how it's made.")

We paused to watch a pair of beefy men wearing what appeared to be long underwear, arms clasped around one another's shoulders, heads squeezed together, slowly circle in the centre of a field ringed with onlookers, until one, attempting to lift the other, slipped and fell onto his back.

"Cumberland wrestling," a white-haired codger leaned over and explained. "Local. *Very* local."

Stewart circulated through the downhome crowd with ease. He can find his footing anywhere. A graduate of Eton and Oxford, he was a summer tutor to princes William and Harry, and became friends with their father. As a member of the British Foreign Office, he was posted to Indonesia to help sort out East Timor, and then to Montenegro during the Kosovo conflict. He served as the deputy governor of two provinces in southern Iraq and ran a charitable foundation in Kabul dedicated to reviving traditional Afghan arts and architecture. Stewart was also a professor of human rights at Harvard and director of the Carr Center for Human Rights Policy at the university's Kennedy School of Government. All before he turned 40.

His public profile is befittingly large. Before he was married, *Vanity Fair* featured him in a list of hot, danger-seeking bachelors, although it also slagged him — wide nose, bushy eyebrows, expressive lips, shaggy hair — as a "dead ringer for one or more of the Rolling Stones." *Esquire* named him one of the 75 most influential people of the 21st century, "because he may be prime minister one day, if he finds it interesting enough." Brad Pitt's production company bought the rights to Stewart's life story and was reported to be developing a biopic, with Orlando Bloom cast in the lead role, although Stewart's gig as a Tory appears to have killed the project. "It's just a phenomenally bad end to a film," he said to the *Guardian*.

"Rory Stewart seems to display a dreamlike disconnection with the world as other mortals experience it," Julian Glover wrote in that newspaper during the 2010 election campaign. "Walking with him, I find myself half-expecting to be beamed back at any moment to his home galaxy."

So he's not your average backbencher. Or your average backpacker. Which fuelled my fascination with his obsessive walking. How deeply did it inform his perspectives? Could it help foster more genuine political engagement? Would he grind my idealistic beliefs into the mud under the boots of worldly realism?

After leaving the Foreign Office, Stewart spent a year and a half walking across the Middle East and Central Asia to Nepal, yet one section was missing from the middle of his journey. So in January 2002, with American and British bombs still echoing, he entered Afghanistan without an entry visa, hoping to embark on a six-week solo march through the mountains, from Herat to Kabul. An enigmatic country viewed as "backward, peripheral, and irrelevant," he writes in his magnificent book, *The Places in Between*, had rocketed into the crosshairs of the world's attention. Stewart felt a need to experience "the place in between the deserts and the Himalayas, between Persian, Hellenic, and Hindu culture, between Islam and Buddhism, between mystical and militant Islam." He wanted to see "where these cultures merged into one another or touched the global world."

Afghanistan's secret police, remarkably efficient just a fortnight into the provisional government, six weeks after the fall of the Taliban, did not think this was such a brilliant idea. "There are three metres of snow on the high passes, there are wolves, and this is war," Stewart was told by an interrogator after being whisked away from his hotel. "You will die, I can guarantee."

The riverside assembly on the Lune adjourns with another round of snickering about salmon sex, and Stewart and I walk downstream along an old farm track. Still in his suit and tightly knotted tie, he deconstructs the meeting. Certainly, it's important to protect the interests of the fishermen, he says. Long a cog in Cumbrian culture, they help safeguard the natural heritage of the area. It's a healthy pastime, and with tackle and restaurant meals rung in, angling adds a few quid to local cash registers. On the other hand, agriculture is the cornerstone of the constituency's financial health, and farmers complain to Stewart about excessive regulations around fertilizer use. Also, he's a proponent of hydro power, because it supplies renewable energy, and he considers it a lesser evil than wind turbines — a source of contentious debate in Cumbria, most of it over their impact on the stunning hill views that propel Lake District tourism. Aquaculture up the coast in Scotland and abnormally heavy rainstorms whipped up by a warming climate make the questions about fishing that much more complex.

"How am I supposed to resolve all of this?" Stewart asks in a gentle voice. "What am I supposed to do?"

He stops to swing open a gate, which protests with a high-pitched squeal, then closes it after we pass through. The meeting with anglers, he says, revealed "only a tiny bit of the river's life" — a glimpse of the specialized issues one must grapple with to attempt a sensible governing stance. "As you begin to talk these things through, you realize what's happening to contemporary societies. We're at these extraordinary impasses," he says, shifting his gaze beyond the Lune. "I believe, because I am a romantic, that it is possible to find solutions. That with enough care, and time and patience, you can come up with the right answer.

"But it doesn't feel like that as a politician. It actually feels, often, as though these things are just conflicts between blind interests which can never be resolved."

Stewart stoops over and plucks a blade of grass from a patch growing beside the hard-packed wheel rut. "We have a problem here," he says, showing me the feathery seed head. This grass needs to be eaten before the seeds develop, otherwise it doesn't deliver enough nutrients to sheep. But farmers have limited stock, so the grass grows ungrazed, and their flocks lose interest. Thistle and nettles sprout and spread, and the amount of edible ground contracts. This leads to higher feed costs, more chemical input and the deterioration of pastureland, to the detriment of farmers, walkers, tourists. It took Stewart three years in office to learn how to read the grass.

At the end of his first summer as an MP, Stewart completed a four-day, 80-mile walk along the River Eden, east of the Lune, from its source to the sea. He was accompanied by the director of Eden Rivers Trust, as well as, during various legs, somebody from Natural England, a representative of the U.K. Environment Agency, a dairy farmer, a fisherman and a biologist, and the trek raised money for a program that brings schoolchildren to the river for environmental education. There were hands-on activities, including a hunt for endangered white-clawed crayfish, the only species native to the British Isles. Shadowed by limestone hills and Roman-era history, the Eden Valley is fertile and green, dotted with oak and chestnut trees. As he walked toward Solway Firth, Stewart absorbed all the information he could about the valley. The dairy farmer, whose family has worked the riverside for centuries, pointed out that the crayfish live only over limestone; they need its calcium for their shells. Another hiker, a medical doctor, showed Stewart the meditation caves that early Christian monks had carved into the cliffs. After four days, stumbling over mud flats at the edge of the sea, Stewart realized how far he had travelled and how much he did not yet understand.

In Afghanistan, despite speaking Dari and some rusty Urdu, despite his experience as a diplomat and as an independent traveller in countries such as Iraq and Iran, that feeling never waned.

The secret police begrudgingly granted him permission to proceed on his walk, though only with two armed escorts. Ragged militias roamed the countryside. A dozen foreign war correspondents had been killed in the previous two months. The men assigned to protect Stewart — Qasim, small and in his mid-40s, and Abdul Haq, taller and younger — were ill-equipped. Mujahidin who had fought against the Russians, and later against the Taliban, now in the employ of a warlord-turned-regional-governor who had done the same, they carried only rifles and sleeping bags, no food or warm clothing. Worse, while agents of the administration in Herat, they had no real authority beyond the Tajik Sunni villages a few days to the east. Travelling with Qasim and Haq was dangerous. On Stewart's route, feudal commanders presided over neighbouring valleys. War had been constant for more than two decades, but the battle lines were seldom clear. There were three other main ethnic groups, another branch of Islam and strongmen who may or may not have been friends with the Taliban just a few short weeks earlier. Some had ties to the Iranian government; others received money and weapons from Pakistan. Alliances give you power in Afghanistan, and they were swinging wildly in the wake of the Western bombardment.

Unwashed, clad in a traditional *shalwar kemis* shirt, baggy pants and a soft, round-topped cap, Stewart could almost pass for a local when he set out from Herat, 60 miles east of the Iranian border. The gravel desert was treeless, flanked by bare hills. The temperature, cool. It felt good to be walking. To satisfy his craving for history and culture and motion.

Securing accommodation each night was an adventure. Muslim tradition holds that travellers must be shown hospitality — "he who sleeps on a full stomach whilst his neighbour goes hungry is not a true believer," proclaimed the Prophet Muhammad — yet the reception varied. Stewart never knew what would happen when he rapped on the door of a mosque or the gate of a walled compound. In some humble mud houses, he was graciously led to the guest room, where he sat on the carpet with men from the village, and after reciting a string of ritual Arabic greetings, fielded questions about his homeland and customs. (*Peace be with you. May you not be tired. I hope your family is well. Would you marry your first cousin?*) Some hosts were suspicious of the foreigner. But Stewart had letters of introduction from high-ranking officials, and most men he encountered were either curious or generous, even if they could not read. Fires were lit, blankets distributed. Meals (rice with a few morsels of mutton for dinner, nan bread and sweet tea for breakfast) were taken in silence. In more prosperous homes, he was served walnuts and oranges by servants while seated on fine carpets. Nowhere was there electricity or indoor plumbing. And until he reached the land of the Hazara, at the midpoint of his walk, there were no women in public. "In many houses," he writes, "the only piece of foreign technology was a Kalashnikov, and the only global brand was Islam."

In one cold, crowded guest room during the first week of the journey, suffering from dysentery and growing weary of the limited conversation, steering clear of religion but willing to dive into politics, Stewart asked a mullah what he thought of Afghanistan's then brand-new leader, Hamid Karzai.

"Good," replied the mullah. "Up till now."

"Up till now?"

"Al-Qaeda was good at the beginning."

Stewart asked another man, a wealthy landowner, why he became a Mujahid.

"Because the Russian government stopped my women from wearing head scarves and confiscated my donkeys."

Why did he fight the Taliban?

"Because they forced my women to wear burkas and stole my donkeys."

Rulers came and went, and it didn't really matter whether they were religious militants or represented foreign superpowers. People had more immediate concerns.

Within a couple of days, Stewart reached the Hari Rud River. In places, it was pinched between terraced hillsides and roared through claustrophobic gorges — prime locations for an ambush. He gave Qasim and Abdul Haq some money and the gunmen agreed to turn back. Once Stewart was alone, villagers would shoulder their Kalashnikovs and insist on guiding him partway to the next cluster of houses. "I was passed like a parcel down the line," he writes, "from one chief to the next."

These chiefs were the only real power. In Afghanistan's tribal mountain villages, people do not pay taxes, nor do they receive anything from the state. Laws are dictated by tradition, religion and necessity. By the land and the seasons. Government happened somewhere else, "in grand bullet-scarred buildings in Herat and Kabul."

In Chaghcharan, a town of 15,000 at the midpoint of his journey, Stewart saw the breadth of the gap between Western rhetoric and Afghan reality. A pair of Chinook helicopters landed and two United

Nations officials ducked out below the whirling blades. An Irishman and a German, they were old hands at international politicking, as knowledgeable about Afghanistan as any European could hope to become. Addressing a crowd from a microphone in front of the town's only concrete building, they explained the new *loya jirga* process that would ultimately select a national leader. Ordinary people, including women, could be nominated as delegates. Then the U.N. men got into the choppers and flew away.

Stewart had friends who worked for the U.N., other international agencies and think tanks in Kabul. They ran projects that cost millions of dollars but rarely left the fortified compounds where they lived. Their goal, he writes, quoting a United Nations document, was "the creation of a centralized, broad-based multiethnic government committed to democracy, human rights, and the rule of law." Regardless of their intentions and sensitivity, they "came from post-modern, secular, globalized states with liberal traditions in law and government." Did they not realize that centralized rule, in this part of the world, usually meant violent subjugation? That democracy and gender equality would not easily find purchase? "Policy-makers," he declares in *The Places in Between*, "did not have the time, structures, or resources for a serious study of an alien culture. They justified their lack of knowledge and experience by focusing on poverty and implying that dramatic cultural differences did not exist."

At a seminar in Kabul, Stewart had listened to Mary Robinson, then the U.N. High Commissioner for Human Rights, remark that Afghan villagers were like poor people the world over — their biggest worry was where their next meal would come from. Yet the peasant farmers he met had a much better idea than most of us about the source of their next meal. Their fields. Their flocks.

You can learn a great deal about an Afghan village very quickly, Stewart says to me as we continue along the Lune. Lives are dramatic. People are literally shooting their neighbours. Or they have run out of food. They will point out bits of local lore: there is where I killed a wolf, there is where I killed a Taliban. Soon after arriving in somebody's home, Stewart would be sitting in a room with a dozen men. They would ask him blunt questions, and half would sleep there with him.

It takes a lot longer to understand a British town, to learn about its problems. People are much more private. They spend more time inside. Farms are larger and pastures are not dotted with shepherds, hollering at you from atop ridges, beckoning you to join them for tea. When he began his campaign hike, Stewart tried to transplant his method from Afghanistan to England. Locals were friendly enough, but not everybody invited him in. "I'd call the police if someone looking like you knocked on my door at night," one friend cautioned. "No one's going to put you up. You'll probably be mugged on the first day. I'd stick to the Taliban."

The contrast is even more striking when it comes to being effective as an administrator or parliamentarian. In 2005, Stewart returned to Afghanistan and lived in Kabul for three years, running the Turquoise Mountain Foundation. While he was there, the charity established a health clinic and primary school, reconstructed 90 buildings and hooked up water and electricity for hundreds of houses. In his first three years of elected office at home, one of his biggest accomplishments has been securing broadband internet access for 52 rural homes — the product of about 120 hours of meetings.

"In a society like this, people have real needs, but they are very complicated to understand," says Stewart. "You wake up some days and you look out the door and things are not too bad. Everybody has a school, everybody has a road, everybody has a water supply, nobody is starving. So what do I really have to do? What's the point of being a politician?

"You can feel very superfluous today," he continues. "You can often feel that all the major problems have been solved. That, basically, we are a society at peace that operates quite well. That I could be knocked over by a bus, and even if they didn't have a Member of Parliament for 20 years, the roads would still be mended, the trains would still run, the electricity would still come. In a mature democracy like this, you need to be very sensitive to minor changes. You have to work more, study more and learn more to squeeze the last bits of use out of what it means to be a public servant."

By walking across domestic and distant landscapes, Rory Stewart has become more intimate with diverse peoples and cultures. He has gained a more nuanced understanding of his constituency, and a war zone, than most politicians will ever obtain. Stewart is far too independent to be allowed near the front bench, says British political writer Ian Dunt. He's probably right. But transformation seldom starts from a seat at the tables of power.

Stewart hiked through Cumbria to capture the attention of its people. Throughout the planet, people walk to capture the attention of politicians. Non-violent civil disobedience is a slow bleed toward change.

Henry David Thoreau wrote one of the movement's founding texts. Motivated by his disgust toward slavery and American imperialism, and briefly jailed for refusing to pay a poll tax, he wrote the essay "Civil Disobedience" in 1849, not long after departing Walden Pond. He called for people to act in accord with their consciences — not to stand back and wait for justice — if they disagreed with a government that purported to be acting on their behalf. Over the next 10 years, Thoreau presented and refined a pair of lectures that evolved into another essay, "Walking," published just after his death from tuberculosis in 1862. It praises the virtues of immersion in nature and condemns private ownership of wilderness. Even a familiar walk, he wrote, can provide new perspectives.

The first global figure to embody Thoreau's words and link civil disobedience with walking in an everlasting way was Mahatma Gandhi. Monopolistic British laws prohibited Indians from producing or selling salt, forcing a mostly poor populace to purchase expensive, often imported salt from their colonizers. In March 1930, Gandhi began a march through the western state of Gujarat, from his ashram to the Arabian Sea. Joined by a few dozen followers at the outset, he spoke at every village where he stopped. Hundreds more joined the procession. On April 5, after nearly 250 miles, he reached the coastal village of Dandi and picked up handfuls of salt from the shore, breaking the law. The protest continued for another two months. Gandhi was arrested in May, inspiring others to lift salt from the sea. By the end of the year, 60,000 people had been thrown in jail, and the journey toward Indian independence was unstoppable.

Notwithstanding recent pedometer counts, Americans are good at making noise with their feet. On March 3, 1913 — the day before the inauguration of President-elect Woodrow Wilson — the Women's Suffrage Parade streamed down Washington's Pennsylvania Avenue, seeking a constitutional amendment that would give women the right to vote. There were 8,000 marchers, 20 floats and nine bands. The route was packed with tens of thousands of spectators, largely men who were in the city for Wilson's ceremony. Female marchers were pushed, tripped and hurt; 100 wound up in the hospital. Policemen did nothing. This became a major news story, and the police superintendent was fired. Wilson's indifference began to erode. Seven years later, the 19th Amendment was passed. Suffering begat suffrage.

Since then, virtually every protest group in the U.S., mainstream and marginal, has taken to the streets of Washington. Fifty thousand Ku Klux Klan members marched along Pennsylvania Avenue in 1925, a ghostly procession of white hoods. Following in their footsteps came rabbis, war veterans, peace activists, feminists, anti-abortion crusaders, farmers, gays and lesbians, trade unionists, environmentalists, Tea Partyers and hundreds of other parties representing the righteous and outraged masses.

On August 28, 1963, Washington prepared for a riot. Four thousand soldiers stood by in the suburbs, and 15,000 paratroopers were on alert in North Carolina. Liquor sales were suspended in D.C. for the first time since Prohibition. Stores shipped away merchandise to prevent looting. At least 250,000 people streamed into the National Mall during the March on Washington for Jobs and Freedom. Joan Baez, Bob Dylan and other musicians performed. The crowd remained peaceful, harmonious — "white legs and negro legs dangle together in the reflecting pool," wrote one reporter. When Martin Luther King, Jr., finally took the microphone at the foot of the Lincoln Memorial, he cast aside his prepared speech. Instead, he preached about his dream of freedom.

"Next to sex, the activity combining bodily experience and intense emotion to the highest degree is the participation in a mass demonstration at a time of great public exaltation," wrote British historian Eric Hobsbawm. "Unlike sex, which is essentially individual, it is by its nature collective . . . and it can be prolonged for hours. . . . It implies some physical action — marching, chanting slogans, singing — through which the merger of the individual in the mass, which is the essence of the collective experience, finds expression."

The March on Washington paved the way to another leap forward. On March 7, 1965, about 600 activists started walking from Selma, Alabama, to Montgomery, the state capital, demanding voting rights and an end to violence and racial discrimination against blacks. They were willing to pass through and camp out in KKK-dominated Lowndes County, where 70 percent of the population was black, though none had tried to vote since 1900. The marchers were beaten back by riot police with nightsticks and tear gas after crossing Selma's main bridge. Two days later, as images of the brutality filtered across the country, King led 2,500 people back to the bridge. They were waiting for a court order that would prevent the police from interfering. When they reached the Alabama River and a cordon of state troopers, they stopped and prayed. The nation held its breath. And then King shouted, "We will go back to the church now." The marchers retreated.

This display of resolve and patience epitomized a "non-violent quest to transform what was normal," civil rights historian Taylor Branch writes in *The King Years: Historic Moments in the Civil Rights Movement*, in which he focuses on this largely forgotten "turnaround march" as one of the era's key moments. On March 21, five days after the retreat, now protected by a federal judge's signature and a couple thousand U.S. Army soldiers, 8,000 people began the 54-mile walk to Montgomery. "My feet felt like they were praying," remarked Rabbi Abraham Heschel. Four days later, at the state capital, King made the speech we know as "How Long, Not Long": "Once more the method of non-violent resistance was unsheathed from its scabbard, and once again an entire community was mobilized to confront the adversary. And again the brutality of a dying order shrieks across the land. Yet, Selma, Alabama, became a shining moment in the conscience of man. . . . If the worst in American life lurked in its dark streets, the best of American instincts arose passionately from across the nation to overcome it."

Indigenous Americans and Canadians continue to march for justice. Although their struggle was already 500 years old, it gained momentum during the civil-rights era. The American Indian Movement advocacy group was formed in 1968. Ten years later, AIM organized a 3,200-mile walk from San Francisco to Washington. It wanted to draw attention to proposed federal legislation that would contravene treaties protecting land and water rights. Twenty-eight people completed the entire five-month trek, enduring blizzards as they crossed the Sierra Nevada mountains and passing through states where they were not permitted to walk on freeways and bridges. In Reno, they were not allowed to use the main street. At the Washington Monument, Prof. Lehman Brightman, a Sioux from South Dakota who in 1969 had established the country's first Native American studies program, at the University of California, Berkeley, spoke of the resources on native land — uranium, coal, oil, gas, timber and water — that the government wanted to steal. "Today's a damn good day," said Brightman, paraphrasing Crazy Horse, "to fight them on this legislation." None of the 11 proposed laws were passed.

In 2000, about 20 Seri and Tohono O'odham Indians from Mexico and the American southwest did the Desert Walk for Biodiversity, Health and Heritage, a 12-day, 230-mile hike from El Desemboque, Mexico, to Tucson, Arizona. They ate only food from the land and learned about "the complex intersections of desert ecology, human health and culture," writes Susie O'Brien, a cultural studies professor at McMaster University in Hamilton, Ontario. It was "an intervention in a struggle for sovereignty over time . . . granting its participants a stake in the promotion of a habitable global future." Their route passed through the hot, dry terrain where thousands of illegal migrants have died attempting to cross into the United States, but the Desert Walk did not focus on immigration policy. It was a protest against the colonization of the future.

Aboriginal history is filled with tales of people who walked great distances to bring about some kind of change, says Leanne Simpson, a scholar and author from the Alderville First Nation, northeast of Toronto. By walking, they could socialize, strengthen family bonds and engage in diplomacy. "The same things that motivated my ancestors to walk," she says, "are motivating people now."

Long marches are much more than a tactic or a strategy, says Simpson, who has taught a course on indigenous resistance at Alberta's Athabasca University. "Indigenous people have long rallied against erasure: erasure from the land, erasure from American and Canadian consciousness. Putting our bodies back on the land can be very powerful."

Canada's Indian Act prevented Aboriginal people from mobilizing in large groups until the 1950s. Revisions loosened the restrictions on public protests, and the walking tradition was reborn. In 1974, the Native Caravan Trek to Ottawa drew activists from across the country, many of whom walked to rallying points before taking a train to the capital to complain about broken treaties. The RCMP, leery of the American Indian Movement and the influence of "radicals" from the U.S., forcibly removed demonstrators from Parliament Hill.

Three years later, Sandra Lovelace, a Maliseet from the Tobique First Nation in New Brunswick, returned to her reserve after getting divorced from her American husband. The homes of relatives were too crowded for Lovelace and her son, but the band council did not help her secure a place to live because she was "non-status" — she had married a white man. Angry that the Indian Act denied her access to her own land and imposed a patriarchal system of identity, Lovelace complained to the United Nations Human Rights Commission. Then, in July 1979, inspired by AIM's trek to Washington, she helped lead the Native Women's Walk to Ottawa.

Lovelace left Tobique on a bus, which stopped at other reserves and picked up more people as it drove west. Just past Montreal, they spent the night on the floor of the town hall in Oka, Quebec, where Mohawk warriors would set up a blockade in 1990. Fifty women and children started walking the next morning. The temperature topped 100° Fahrenheit, feet and ankles ached, but communities on the route provided cold water, sandwiches and places to sleep. National media picked up the story; politicians, both federal and Aboriginal, met with the walkers. Seven days and 100 miles later, they marched through a crowd to the steps of Parliament Hill. Prime Minister Joe Clark promised that the Indian Act would be revised, and in 1985 the status law for women was finally changed.

"We really didn't think anybody would listen to us, or that we would accomplish anything," says Lovelace, who became Canada's first female Aboriginal senator in 2005. "Just getting there was emotional."

In the last few years, Aboriginal women have walked across hundreds of miles of Arctic ice to raise money to fight cancer, and along British Columbia's "Highway of Tears," where dozens of young women, almost all Aboriginal, have been murdered or gone missing. Josephine Mandamin, an Anishinabe elder from northern Ontario, led a series of long walks along the shorelines of the Great Lakes. She grew up drinking water straight from Georgian Bay and eating fresh fish every day. To her, pollution and global warming are no abstraction. "First Nations' grandmothers do not love their grandkids more than you love yours," says Kevin McMahon, director of the documentary film *Waterlife*, which features Mandamin, "but they may have a clearer view of the horizon."

The Indian Act remains a lightning rod. It perpetuates paternalism and racism, says Leo Baskatawang, an Anishinabe from northern Ontario. In the summer of 2012, while working toward a master's degree in Native studies, he chained a copy of the Act to his leg and walked from Vancouver to Ottawa. Averaging around 20 miles a day along the Trans-Canada Highway, he wore through 40 copies of the legislation. "These types of walks, they're not exclusively indigenous things," says Baskatawang, who didn't do much walking until going on a pair of tours of Iraq as a soldier in the U.S. Army. His biggest inspiration was Terry Fox, who ran halfway across Canada on one leg in 1980 to convince people to support cancer research. Similarly, Baskatawang says that his walk "was a way to share my message with a lot of people over an extended period of time. If you want to see change happen, you have to go out and actively seek it."

Stanley Vollant feels the same way about the Indian Act, but Innu Meshkenu is focused on individual healing and community strength. He looks at politics through a wide-angle lens. When I asked him about Canada's governing party, he took me on a long tangent, all the way back to the Battle of Marathon, in 490 BC, when the Greeks triumphed against a much larger Persian army. Then he told me that he has been asked to run for office by the federal New Democrats and Quebec's Liberals. Although he has his eyes on a health minister's portfolio, he is a decade away from even considering such a move. "For me, it's important to finish things before starting new ones," said Vollant. "Finishing these walks will give me better knowledge of my country, of my people and of the real challenges people are facing."

In February 2013, as I prepared to travel to Manawan for the expedition with Vollant, hereditary chief Beau Dick of the Namgis First Nation led a nine-day walk from Alert Bay, British Columbia, to the provincial capital building in Victoria. The march down Vancouver Island was part of the Idle No More protest movement. Chief Dick wanted to raise awareness about proposed federal legislation, Bill C-38, an omnibus act that contained a couple hundred pages of amendments that would weaken Canada's environmental laws.

As the group approached Victoria, its ranks swelled from a few dozen to several hundred. City councillor Ben Isitt joined for the final half-dozen miles. The conversations he had while walking for two hours were meaningful. Businesspeople know how to build relationships and partnerships on the golf course. Informal mixing on a march or a picket line, says Isitt, encourages solidarity and helps activists pursue goals collectively.

Before being elected to municipal office, Isitt wrote and lectured about history at universities in British Columbia and New Brunswick, where his PhD thesis focused on the working class and political change. When I ask about the historical union between walking and civil disobedience, Isitt tells me about one of the longest protest marches on B.C. soil. In the 1950s, in the Kootenay Mountains, the Sons of Freedom — a radical splinter branch of the pacifist Christian Doukhobor sect — pulled their children from public schools they deemed militaristic and materialistic. Kids were forcibly rounded up by the government and interned at residential schools. Some of their families responded by bombing a courthouse, an electricity transmission tower, railway bridges and tracks, and setting schools on fire. More than 100 people were eventually convicted of these crimes and, in the spring of 1962, incarcerated in a new, fireproof, purpose-built, maximum-security prison in Agassiz, east of Vancouver on the Fraser River.

That September, roughly 600 Freedomite men, women and children began a march-cum-migration from the Kootenays to Vancouver and, the following summer, to the gates of the prison, where they established an encampment. Agassiz residents had mixed reactions to their new neighbours. Some (grocers, the pharmacist) welcomed the business; others were hostile. The RCMP kept a respectful watch. Health inspectors were satisfied with the camp's sanitary conditions. Freedomite kids attended local schools, where they were excused from singing patriotic songs in recognition of their religious convictions. Men worked for nearby farmers or built and painted houses. No longer hidden away in the secluded valleys of the B.C. Interior, the migration brought the Sons of Freedom (and, more broadly, the entire Doukhobor sect) into the public consciousness. The tent village lasted for nearly a decade, until all of the inmates had served their time. When they were released, the Freedomites returned home and the simmering tensions faded. An understanding — and an enduring peace — had been struck.

Walking a long distance for a purpose instead of taking a bus or car has symbolic power, says Isitt. Travelling along major transportation routes and passing through communities can capture the public's attention in ways that other protests might not. These marches belong to a spectrum that also includes funeral processions and parades, which can be political or celebratory, or somewhere in between. A gay pride march in one city might be festive, while in an another city it could be angry and defiant. Regardless, it is an elemental way to close the gap, physically and metaphorically, between where you are and where you want to be.

Governments are large, lumbering ships. They seldom alter course quickly. Individual or group actions can nudge policy in one direction or another. But even if there's a convincing case to be made — say, the wide-ranging rewards of a particular mode of locomotion — the bureaucratic or partisan (or vested-interest) heel-dragging can be infuriating, as University of Regina climate-change researcher Dave Sauchyn was rudely reminded.

A dedicated walker who moved farther from campus so he could enjoy a longer commute on foot, Sauchyn revels in the hostility with which Regina treats pedestrians: streets with no sidewalks or crosswalks; cul-de-sacs that impede direct routes. He has knocked on front doors and asked to cut through backyards. "People stare at me," he says. "They think I'm unemployed, homeless or mentally ill."

As a member of the Prairie Adaptation Research Collaborative, Sauchyn was asked to speak in front of the federal government's Standing Committee on Environment and Sustainable Development. Encouraged not to deliver a dry, scientific talk, he penned a preamble about walking. "I began my remarks by suggesting that two of Parliament's most challenging issues, health care and the environment, could be addressed with a single solution: encouraging Canadians to walk," says Sauchyn. "This suggestion was met with spontaneous laughter and a second round of chuckles when one MP noted that I live in Regina. I suppose they misinterpreted my sincere advice as an attempt to preface my talk with some humour."

Sauchyn's research is technical. He studies how watersheds have responded to climactic changes over the past millennium. His pie charts are not uplifting. Some days, especially after talking to business associations or politicians, he is cynical. Other times, when he is with farmers or ranchers or people who are close to the land, he is more optimistic. He draws inspiration from local accomplishments and feels a responsibility to deliver a personal message: "We need lifestyles compatible with alleviating the effects of global warming. Anything that represents a shift in attitude, a shift away from car culture, represents adaptation to or mitigation against climate change."

Urging people to walk is not the federal government's responsibility, Sauchyn knows. The creation of walkable communities is mostly municipal terrain. Regina, despite its reputation for winters as inhospitable as Edmonton's, is improving. Before she became Toronto's chief planner, Jennifer Keesmaat was a consultant with a firm hired to develop a plan for the city's downtown neighbourhoods. She titled the document "Walk to Work." Released in 2009, it called for 5,000 new downtown residents over 15 years: a population base of young professionals, artists, students, seniors and families that would support niche retail in a city experiencing unprecedented growth. If Regina follows her recommendations, people will be walking to work along streets designed for pedestrians — streets with the type of friendly facades, transit links, parks and gathering places that Jeff Speck applauds in *Walkable City*.

Since 1986, when Regina's previous downtown plan was created, the city had made minimal investments in public spaces. It wasn't unusual for a heritage building to be torn down to make way for a parking lot, even though parking lots covered more than one-quarter of all downtown real estate. This approach did not foster a critical mass of restaurants, shops, galleries and performance halls that would keep people in the urban core after dark. And it's those people who make a downtown lively and safe.

Keesmaat's plan was approved by Regina city council in 2012, but already a pair of major new buildings (an office tower and a condo high-rise) had been designed to include public plazas, street furniture and awnings that will mitigate the concrete-canyon wind-tunnel effect. The city has implemented less restrictive sidewalk-café guidelines and halted the expansion of its network of elevated pedways between buildings, because they remove people from the street. "The last time something like this happened with our down-town, it was 20 years ago," Regina's mayor said in a radio interview, "so we wanted to make sure we got it right."

Canada's provincial governments also have a horse in this race. In Ontario, where the annual health-care bill is about $50 billion, the Ministry of Health promotes walking as a way to counter obesity, diabetes, cancers and dozens of other physical and mental ailments. The Ministry of Municipal Affairs and Housing supports the development of mixed-use neighbourhoods that increase rates of active transportation. "Community design," states its land-use planning handbook, "influences how people travel and how physically active they are in the course of the day." Metrolinx, the provincial agency created to coordinate and integrate all transportation in the greater Toronto and Hamilton area, one of the fastest-growing regions in the country, envisions safe and convenient pedestrian access to a network of mobility hubs where buses and trains connect. The Ministry of Infrastructure sees walking and cycling as an everyday element of urban transportation.

This policy work is the domain of the public service. It trickles into our lives slowly. You don't hear heated debates about walking in the provincial legislature — it's not a campaign flashpoint. But that didn't deter my one-track mind when I saw John Fraser striding toward my driveway.

I was in the back of my van, packing for a camping trip. There was a by-election coming up in my riding. Liberal leader and premier Dalton McGuinty had stepped down, and Fraser, the premier's right-hand man, was hoping to step up.

"You're busy," he said, seeing me wrestle with sleeping bags and plastic bins crammed with rain gear. "I won't stay long."

"No, please," I said, jumping out of the van. "I've got time."

A large man with a bushy swoosh of grey hair, John Kerry meets Jay Leno, Fraser told me about his career in the grocery business, and how he took a "temporary" leave of absence to work with McGuinty 18 years earlier. He asked for my support and promised to continue serving the residents of Ottawa South.

"So," I said when he had finished his spiel, "are you doing a lot of door-knocking?"

"Seven days a week," said Fraser. "I've lost 16 pounds so far. My knees are giving me problems, though. I came in too heavy, too hard. I've started to see a physiotherapist."

I explained why I was curious about canvassing, and he said he had been doing it for years, with McGuinty and other politicians. "I'll tell you one thing — it feels totally different when you're the candidate.

"And you know what?" he added. "If more people walked, the world would be a better place."

Fraser invited me to join him on the campaign trail. A couple of weeks later, I met him and five young volunteers on a residential street not far from my house. Fraser and the Conservative candidate were even in the polls, and the election was five days away.

"How was that camping trip?" he asked, exhibiting door-knocking strategy number one: learn something about each person you shake hands with, and remember it. His job out here, essentially, is to show constituents that if they need help, he will be approachable. "There is genuine skepticism about the political process," he said. In a single day, when every tweet and Facebook post is tabulated, candidates receive the same amount of media coverage that would have taken them six months to accumulate 30 years ago. This has a desensitizing effect. Voters are busy; you need to find a way to connect. "This is exactly how you win elections — by walking," Fraser's campaign manager, Jackie Choquette, had told me. "Nothing replaces that door-to-door interaction."

Fraser pulled a small bottle of mouthwash out of his pocket, swished it around, then spit into a sewer drain. Garlicky shawarma had been on the menu at the campaign office. Cradling clipboards that indicated where undecided voters lived, the volunteers fanned out. Fraser had a list of addresses to try. He knocked on a screen door and a white-haired woman answered. He introduced himself; she was in the middle of cooking dinner. "I just want to tell you one thing," Fraser told her. "I love what I do and I believe I can make a difference."

For the next hour, he knocked on doors and asked residents about their concerns. Homecare for seniors. Youth jobs. Hospital funding. Fraser spoke knowledgeably about all of these issues. While working behind the scenes for the premier, he was the riding's de facto MPP. He knows what to say and when to say it (such as his remark, within minutes of meeting me, that walking can make the world a better place). Only once, when a woman started talking about a private-home day-care task force she was on, did he seem anxious to get moving. The clock was ticking. There were 80,000 voters to visit and the campaign was only seven weeks long. "It's important to remember," he told me as we approached the next house, "that the smartest person in the room knows what they don't know."

It was a muggy evening. Dark clouds rolled in. The sky darkened. Thunder roared. Raindrops started falling. Fraser and the volunteers walked quickly back to their van. "Who wants ice cream?" he asked. "Let's go get ice cream. We can wait this out."

"In any country, politicians are the lowest form of life," Rory Stewart said to me as we were leaving the Penrith Show, en route to the River Lune. "But you have to sacrifice yourself on the altar of democracy."

Stewart is leading "one of the most remarkable lives on record," opined the *New York Times*. He is a dreamer, less bound by convention than virtually all of his peers. But his remark that every major problem has been solved was tongue-in-cheek. A juxtaposition of pastoral Cumbria and war-ravaged Afghanistan. Whenever war or extremist violence flares up in a country like Iraq or Syria, whenever jihadists from Western countries make headlines, he is a frequent commentator on current affairs programs and in the op-ed pages, stressing the need for "detailed experience in a particular place," and urging humility and restraint when considering foreign intervention. Thinking beyond the next election, striving for a deep read on the land, surely he can hear the tension building in the connective tissues spidering throughout the globe.

As we huddled behind a stone wall to escape the wind and eat sandwiches on top of the Merrick, Joseph Murphy had told me about the Dark Mountain Manifesto. In 2009, a group of writers and artists in Oxford published a pamphlet warning of "ecological collapse, material contraction and social and political unravelling." They argue that "politics as we have known it totters, like the machine it was built to sustain." Solutions proposed by government and corporate leaders, which usually involve "the necessity of urgent political agreement and a judicious application of human technological genius," are a smokescreen. "Centuries of hubris block our ears like wax plugs; we cannot hear the message which reality is screaming at us." On the precipice of a transformation so colossal we cannot comprehend its scale, the manifesto advises us to look down. To look at the land. At ourselves. At the now. Temporal awareness as an act of resistance.

On our way back to Old Tebay Bridge, Stewart stops and leans against a fence. The Lune burbles behind him. In the modern world, he says, one of the great privileges for a walker is to arrive in a place that has no roads. To reach a community where people ask where you came from, where you are grateful for the right to travel on their land.

He points to the east, a sea of green. "My constituency ends on the top of that hill there." He points to the west. "And on top of that hill there.

"If you climbed that large hill," he continues, pointing south, "you would see my constituency and nothing else, rimmed by the horizon. I feel very lucky to have a home like this. A place with limits and bounds."

Then he tells me about his favourite night of the election campaign hike. It was in the town of Wigton, near the border with Scotland, at a public housing estate with about 150 homes. There is a high unemployment rate in the neighbourhood, a high incidence of drug abuse. One in five people have been in jail. Yet when he crisscrossed its laneways and alleys for six hours with a local, meeting dozens of adults and children, listening to their stories, and then slept on a couch in a flat where three generations of the same family live, he was moved. "I left so joyful and positive, so convinced that it's the most wonderful community," he says. "That's probably a *misleading* sense of things. There are many things there that are very miserable.

"I do believe strongly that in developed countries, in North America and Europe, walking is changing from what it used to be. You need a lot of very thoughtful and original approaches — going to the same place twice, being careful about how you present yourself, travelling with a local — to learn from the experience. You have to work harder than you do walking across Afghanistan.

"My dream," he continues, "would be to be able to take a year off to walk through Cumbria and spend time in every village, meeting *everybody*. As a Member of Parliament, I want to learn more. But I think my constituents would get fed up if I took a year off to go wandering."

six

CREATIVITY

"Walking exposes us to the constant flux of a changing environment, providing us with an endless array of new and unique experiences, which combined with our past memories may, through serendipity alone, provoke new associations and give birth to new ideas."

— *Paul Sowden, psychologist,*
University of Surrey, England

"I can only meditate when I am walking. When I stop, I cease to think; my mind works only with my legs."

— *Jean-Jacques Rousseau,* Confessions

I am descending a long concrete staircase. Backwards. Arm-in-arm with a woman I met half an hour ago. The steps are crowded by creeping shrubs and slick with rain.

In the 1860s, nearly 600 acres of glacier-scoured Brooklyn were transformed into a park by landscape architects Frederick Law Olmsted and Calvert Vaux, better known for their work on a larger rectangle of real estate in the middle of Manhattan a decade earlier. Brooklyn's Prospect Park was created to serve as a green respite in the rapidly growing borough. This staircase leads to the Concert Grove, one of many features designed to blend natural beauty with the recreational facilities sought by residents on this side of the river.

My partner and I feel each step with our toes before dropping downward. We reach the bottom, unlink our arms, pivot 180 degrees in sync and face straight ahead, hands extended toward the sky. Eight other new acquaintances clap and cheer. We are art.

Sheltered under a black umbrella, our curator for the evening, Todd Shalom, lights a cigarette. "Don't worry," he tells his associate, Ben Weber, "we have liability."

Following some gentle directions from Shalom, we line up single-file behind a woman holding a black-and-white umbrella that looks like half a soccer ball. She pirouettes along a maple-and-oak-lined cobblestone path and the rest of us trail behind, mimicking her movements as accurately as possible. We enter a large, open-air octagonal pavilion, where a dozen men are doing capoeira. Weber divides our group into two. Half of us compose a Twisterlike sculpture with our bodies: crouching, arching, shins braced against one another for balance. Our form mirrors the cast-iron columns and oriental cupola of the pavilion. We remain still for a minute. The others then "edit" our poses, repositioning arms and legs until they are satisfied with the configuration. Outstretched limbs and angled torsos now reflect the capoeira swoops and lunges on the far side of the structure.

It is my first trip to Prospect Park, which is across the street from the apartment my grandparents and mother settled in after immigrating to the United States in the early 1960s. I am standing on one foot, eyes closed, hand on a stranger's shoulder, wondering whether my grandfather ever hid from the rain under this roof. Listening to the muffled sounds of traffic, buffered by Brooklyn's only remaining indigenous forest, I can hear Shalom's voice in my head: "The intention is to show someone a new perspective of their environment. We want to encourage an ongoing poetic exchange with the places that people live in and visit."

Shalom, who is wearing skinny jeans and shiny sneakers with bright yellow laces, started organizing participatory art walks in 2004. He grew up in suburban New Jersey, graduated from Boston University with a business degree, then decamped to San Francisco to attend art school and write poems. The walks were a way to take his words off the page, to break down the barriers between artist and audience, to attain the heightened awareness of travel without leaving town. After experimenting with soundscape installations, moving to Buenos Aires, and having a flash of heady clarity while suffering from altitude sickness in Peru, he decided to simplify his work. Shalom stopped fiddling around with ultrasonic sensors and computer coding, landed in Brooklyn and in 2010 launched a collective called Elastic City, whose programming consists of a series of low-fi walks led by artists. "I got frustrated with technology," he says. "I wanted to see what I could do just with my body and a group of people outside."

Although tourists regularly sign up for Elastic City outings, these are not conventional tours, which to Shalom typically "retell somebody's or some group's past experience through data and facts." Instead, the walks — or "ways," as he likes to call them — are a pliable canvas, striving for "a more embodied experience in the present moment." They spark contemplation, fluidity, and a loose choreography among strangers. They encourage adults to see the everyday with the wide-open eyes of a child. To try new things.

I do not enjoy being on display. Karaoke and dancing make me queasy. So I feel a little uncomfortable in the Prospect Park pavilion. This is how Shalom expects people to react. A lot of us are intimidated by participation. But when you're on a walk, you're already moving. The participation is built-in. It's almost a trick, he says. A way to overcome the internal calibrations and cultural expectations that steer us toward the path of least resistance. Walking puts the mind in what French philosopher Frédéric Gros calls a state of "suspensive freedom." And when there is a lightness in your step, thoughts can wander.

On this wet June evening — after my weekend with the Philadelphia police and before my day in Harlem with Matt Green — I have joined Elastic City's Signature Walk, a "greatest hits" compilation of physical, aural and textual play. Other walks focus on sound, sun, shadows or specific locations in New York, both outdoors (the "privatized space" around the exterior of the Lincoln Center) and inside (Grand Central Station).

We leave the pavilion and head to Ocean Avenue, a busy road that borders the park. Shalom instructs us to look for an interesting object and, when ready, to place it on the sidewalk. "If you need it," he says, "we have hand sanitizer."

I snap an ear of reddish fungus off a nearby stump. My collaborators come back with a double-headed mushroom, green and brown leaves, the eraser end of a broken pencil, a candy wrapper, a bottle cap and an orange peel. One by one, we position our finds on the ground. "Okay," says Shalom, "now everybody can move an item, and it doesn't have to be the thing you contributed." After an hour together, nobody is shy about imposing his or her aesthetic. At a glance, our one-square-foot tableau, some objects stacked, others on their own, looks like a random assemblage. Only a closer inspection reveals imagination and intent.

The interplay between walking and new ideas has captivated artists, writers and thinkers since our dawn as a sentient species. In ancient Athens, Aristotle walked back and forth while lecturing at the Lyceum. His followers were known as peripatetics, derived from the Greek word *pateo*, to walk. Another Greek philosopher, Diogenes, gave us the compact expression *solvitur ambulando* — it is solved by walking. Sigmund Freud mapped out the structure of the psyche during long mountain hikes. *The Interpretation of Dreams* "was designed to have the effect of one of his hikes through a concealed pass in a dark forest," writes Michael Michalko, "until it opens out on a view of the plain."

In the late 18th century, from his cottage in England's Lake District, just west of Penrith, William Wordsworth pushed off on ambulatory adventures that ultimately totalled some 180,000 miles. He went on long, meditative walks, with his sister Dorothy or "lonely as a cloud," and wrote the lyrical verse that helped introduce the Romantic Age of English literature, a response to the Industrial Revolution and the aristocratic political and social norms of the era. "By being forced to focus on quick-passing logistical realities such as stepping over uneven ground, the brain is freed up from having to contemplate background worries," Trina-Marie Baird writes in an essay about Wordsworth, "which are both more tedious and less specific than the ground underfoot. . . . Like an LP needle, [the mind] has been lifted up off its original track, and is now free to land along a new groove of its own choosing."

During the same period, in East Prussia, suffering from weak health, Immanuel Kant went for a walk around the university city of Königsberg every day after lunch. "It was arranged with such regularity," reports the *Encyclopedia Britannica*, "that people set their clocks according to his daily walk." In Switzerland a century later, Friedrich Nietzsche maintained an equally disciplined schedule. He worked from dawn until 11 a.m. every morning, then went for a brisk two-hour walk through the forest or along the lakeshore. In *Twilight of the Idols*, Nietzsche wrote that "only thoughts reached by walking have value."

With all due respect to the great philosophers and poets, however, I'm more interested in what walking can reveal about our own little niche in the Anthropocene, what today's creative vanguard is seeing.

In June 1967, a 22-year-old English art student named Richard Long took a train southeast from London's Waterloo Station. He disembarked after 20 miles, found a featureless field edged by tall trees and walked back and forth in a straight line on the grass until his trodden path was clearly visible. Then he took a black-and-white photograph: a vertical whitish stripe through the middle of the bristly field, bushy trees in the background. The image, 14.8 by 12.8 inches, on an off-white paper mount, stands as a key early work in a long and fertile career that revolves exclusively around walking.

"Nature has always been recorded by artists, from prehistoric cave paintings to 20th-century landscape photography. I too wanted to make nature the subject of my work, but in new ways," says Long, who has staged dozens of solo exhibitions throughout the world, from New York's Museum of Modern Art to the Guggenheim in Bilbao, Spain, and has been nominated for Britain's Turner Prize four times, winning the country's most prestigious art award in 1989 for his overall body of work. "I started working outside using natural materials like grass and water," he says, "and this evolved into the idea of making a sculpture by walking. . . . My intention was to make a new art which was also a new way of walking."

Long wanted to borrow the land, but not possess it. His breakthrough photograph, "A Line Made by Walking," was eventually acquired by the Tate Gallery. The "seemingly simple and prosaic action" of trampling a trail through the grass had come to be seen as "dematerialized" art. It was impermanent, ephemeral, humble. It critiqued the materialism of consumer society, circumvented the art market and anticipated the explosion of performance art in the 1970s, according to the Tate catalogue. "Long changed our notion of sculpture and gave new meaning to an activity as old as man himself," wrote gallery director Nicholas Serota. "Nothing in the history of art quite prepared us for the originality of his action."

In July 2013, I took a train north from London to find out what all the fuss was about. An unprecedented international retrospective, *Walk On: From Richard Long to Janet Cardiff — 40 Years of Art Walking*, had just opened at a gallery in Sunderland, a small coastal city east of Newcastle, and one of its curators offered to show me around.

My nose for fine art is not what you would call refined. Whenever I go to a gallery, a scene from the film *L.A. Story* comes to mind. The camera zooms in on Steve Martin as he interprets an off-screen painting to three stone-faced companions. "The way he's holding her, it's almost filthy," Martin says, rhapsodically describing how the artist has captured an imminent kiss, a tangle of legs, breasts beneath a translucent blouse and voyeuristic onlookers lurking behind a door. "I must admit, when I see a painting like this," he says, finishing with vigour, "I get emotionally . . . *erect!*" The camera angle flips to show the canvas: a blotchy red rectangle.

Writing about art is like dancing about architecture, to paraphrase that frequently paraphrased line. Still, I immersed myself in essays about Long and his peers while en route to Newcastle.

Long and Hamish Fulton, his classmate at Saint Martin's School of Art in London from 1966 to 1968, are the two most renowned walking artists on the planet. It's a surprisingly large field. Dozens of others mine walking deeply in their work, but all of the art made by these two men is derived from this basic activity. Long and Fulton have been associated with the wider land-art movement, a form inextricably rooted in nature that emerged in the U.S. in the late 1960s as a protest against the commercialization and artificiality of art. But both reject this characterization. Land art often entails significant alterations to the landscape. (One of the movement's founding creations is American sculptor Robert Smithson's "Spiral Jetty," a 1,500-foot-long, 15-foot-wide coil jutting out from the shore of Utah's Great Salt Lake that he constructed over six days using two dump trucks, a tractor, a front-end loader and 6,650 tons of rock and earth.) Like most of Long's oeuvre, Fulton's art is transient. And though they have walked side by side, a fundamental distinction can be made.

Long is known for embarking on epic walks: 24 hours without stopping, a few days, several weeks. Sometimes he arranges stones, slate, driftwood and other natural objects into lines, circles or spirals, and then photographs the roughly hewn forms. Sometimes he ships the materials back to his studio or a gallery and assembles sculptures. He also makes large-format typographic pieces, such as the wall-sized "Anywhere," which lists in red block letters the things he encountered during an 11-day winter walk in England: roads, footpaths, stones, rivers, stars, mist, dawn, dusk, rain, animal tracks, springs, camps, bones, cairns, footprints, birdsong, flowers, clouds, water, wind, summit, horizons, full moon, the kindness of strangers. Simple things rendered sacred, celebrated for what they are, rather than what we do to or with them.

Long has travelled throughout the globe, from the U.K. and Europe to the Andes, Asia, Africa and the fringes of North America. He has tremendous stamina (walking 82 miles in 24 hours) and has made some technically complex pieces, including "Spring Circle," a ring of blue-green slate, cut from a quarry in Cornwall, England, that was once the deepest man-made pit in the world. Laid on the floor of a gallery in a circle with a ten-foot diameter, smooth on top and around the perimeter but jagged in the middle, the work has its own "internal horizon line, craggy and rugged, pointing perhaps to its source," writes art critic Dorothy Feaver. "Removed from the landscape to the 'white cube' of the gallery space, 'Spring Circle' has a certain autonomy of time and place."

Hamish Fulton never brings materials home. Nor does he leave anything behind. He makes no formal mark on the landscape. Since the late 1960s, he has gone on a series of often multi-day or multi-week walks, in the American West, the Nepalese Himalayas, and more than 20 other countries. His art, channelling mountaineering culture, Buddhism and American Indian spirituality, consists mostly of photography and painted or printed typography. The text is usually minimal, and most walks are recorded by a single image. Instead of literally or liberally documenting a trek, he distills the experience to its essence and then amplifies the scale by blowing up visuals and texts to the size of a wall. "Rock Fall Echo Dust" — 16 letters set in a four-by-four grid, the four words in alternating black and orange sans serif on a pale pink backdrop — has only a shard of context running across the bottom of the canvas: "A twelve and a half day walk on Baffin Island Arctic Canada Summer 1988." Another symmetrical grid of words, "Water Paths River Tides," condenses his six-day walk along the River Thames from source to sea. These minimalist interpretations leave space for audiences to reminisce about their own walks, perhaps — to reconnect with their own experiences in the natural world.

In recent years, Fulton has experimented with format. He made a rare film for a 2012 solo exhibition at the Turner Contemporary gallery in the holiday town of Margate, on the English Channel north of Dover. For "Walk 2: Margate Sands," hundreds of people walked around the concrete perimeter of a rectangular tidal bathing pool on the town's beach. In the close-up half of the split-screen video, the walkers look like marching soldiers. But from a distance, on the other half of the screen, they do not appear to be moving, "as if the pool is edged with a dark blanket-stitch," writes art critic Laura Cumming, "a walking definition of humanity."

Fulton orchestrated another performance piece before his exhibition opened at the Turner. "Slowalk (In support of Ai Weiwei)" brought together 100 people in the cavernous Turbine Hall at the Tate Modern gallery in London, where Weiwei's installation "Sunflower Seeds" — millions of intricately handcrafted porcelain sunflower seeds, tiny symbols of individuality and mass manufacturing — was on display. The Chinese artist, architect and activist had just been arrested in Beijing; his whereabouts were unknown. Fulton asked participants to line the edge of a large open rectangle on the gallery floor, to pick a point somewhere on each of the four sides and to walk slowly to each location for half an hour, returning to their original positions after two hours. A gong was struck and they started walking. When they finished, the gong was struck again and, as Fulton says, "all the particles, the human beings, they all dispersed."

"Only art resulting from the experience of individual walks" is how he describes his work. It is "a passive protest against urban societies that alienate people from the world of nature."

Mike Collier, a 59-year-old Liverpudlian with a greying ponytail, picks me up at the train station near the River Tyne in downtown Newcastle. England's northeast, like Glasgow, is in a post-industrial fog. Shipbuilding, coal mining and other heavy industries have dwindled or vanished, leaving behind a shaky economy built around service and retail jobs. But the region is a decent place to be an artist,

Collier says as he drives toward Sunderland, 15 miles to the east. Rents drop this far from London, and there is less desire for validation from the core.

The University of Sunderland, where Collier is a professor, helps to foster an egalitarian ethic. It's a former polytechnic college with a non-elitist approach to education. In a country with a rigid class system, where universities increasingly focus on STEM subjects (science, technology, engineering and math), where austerity measures have forced arts and environment organizations to compete for increasingly limited funding, this is a busy perch. In addition to lecturing, supervising graduate students, co-curating *Walk On* and helming the university's Walking, Art, Landskip and Knowledge (WALK) research group — a "custodian and critical friend for the practice of art walking" that he established with a pair of academic colleagues — Collier maintains his own studio. Inspired by Wordsworth and 17th-century Japanese haiku master Matsuo Basho, both of whom radically explored our relationship to the natural world using everyday words, he is passionate about the colloquial names of flora and fauna. Collier walks through the hills and along the rivers of England and Scotland, then makes pastel-on-canvas pieces, often dominated by text and blocks of vivid colour. He names the plants and animals he has seen using vanishing folkloric terminology (Lymptwigg, Huggaback) and chooses a representational palette that recreates the emotional experience of the hike, not the static perspective offered by a traditional landscape painting. His resuscitation of lost language shows a conservationist spirit, a veneration of the unheeded diversity underfoot.

"If art is about anything," says Collier, parking on a side street in downtown Sunderland, "it's about people making sense of how they see the world and mediating that experience so that other people can become engaged with it. And one of the simplest things we do, one of the simplest ways we see the world, is by walking through it. Walking gives us time to become engaged with things. It allows all the senses to become engaged."

When I confess that my art vocabulary is rudimentary, Collier promises to help me navigate his exhibition. Walkers have an affinity for each other, he reminds me, just like motorcyclists: "If you break down beside the road, there's always someone there to help."

Before entering the Northern Gallery for Contemporary Art, on the top floor of a municipal building, visitors are greeted by several soundscapes created by Janet Cardiff, who lives in British Columbia and Berlin and is one of Canada's most accomplished contemporary artists. I put on a pair of headphones and listen to "Jena Walk (Memory Field)," an audio piece by Cardiff and her partner George Bures Miller, commissioned by the eastern German city of Jena, where Napoleon fought the Prussians in the early 1800s and where Russian tanks rolled through the mud at the end of World War II. I hear the sounds of 19th-century battle: cannons and muskets firing, horses galloping past. Over top, a woman reads excerpts from the diary of Louise Seidler, a painter from Jena and a friend (and next-door neighbour) of Goethe. Meant to be listened to on location, the binaural recording carries me far from Sunderland. "A walk is an act of contemplation," reads the artist's statement, and this layered narrative "deals with the physicality of memory. . . . Time slips from one century to another as the listener walks, aware of their feet on the earth and the wind on their face. They . . . are walking on the site just as others have walked over the same earth the last two hundred years, their stories mixing with those in the past."

Inside the gallery, most of the floor in the first room is cordoned off for Richard Long's "Fourteen Stones." The installation consists of 14 light brown and pale orange stones, ranging from thigh- to foot-sized, collected from a beach near his home in Bristol. When he first assembled the sculpture, in 1977, it was a circle. Here, the stones resemble the constellation Orion: a stick figure with legs splayed and arms extended. It does not inflame my emotions.

Then I spot one of Long's classics, "England 1968," on the wall. He made it by walking an X into a field of daisies and taking a black-and-white photograph. Once the flowers grew again, his path vanished. One of my daughters is named Daisy, and the picture triggers a memory of her first steps outdoors, on the sidewalk in front of our home in Edmonton. In the pale light of a prairie spring evening, Daisy and her sister Maggie would totter past the neighbour's house and to the corner, yelping gleefully, and then stop and stare wide-eyed at the world beyond the curb. Preserved on digital video, it is time suspended.

Walk On features the work of 37 artists, and when Collier leaves me alone to wander through, Steve Martin slips out of the gallery. The films of Francis Alÿs mesmerize me. A Belgian-born architect who moved to Mexico City, Alÿs is preoccupied with surveillance culture. In "Guards," a 27-minute video, 64 Coldstream Guards, wearing their iconic scarlet tunics and black bearskin hats, separately enter the mostly empty streets of central London. Following a set of prearranged instructions, each guard wanders around on his own until encountering a fellow solider. When two meet, they fall into step together and march as a pair until spotting another guard, who then joins them. Eventually, all 64 are together, marching in an eight-by-eight grid. The video splices together footage of guards — rifles on their shoulders, arms swinging at their sides, boots clacking on pavement — with shots from the point of view of somebody who is walking. Watching it feels like spying on a psychogeographic patrol.

British artist Tim Knowles makes films using a ski helmet with a camera on its side. The helmet is topped by a pivoting kite-like weathervane, and he let the wind guide him around the streets of London in the middle of the night. Blown about like a stray piece of newspaper, the breeze sends him into construction fences and scurrying around Trafalgar Square. Knowles' "Windwalk" features video, photography and, mounted on the wall, the Terry Gilliamesque headgear, as well as a line drawing made using the walk's GPS trail — "charting one man's lonely and often whimsical relationship with the natural world," reads a review in the *Guardian*.

Sarah Cullen, who splits her time between Toronto and London, rigged up a low-tech recording device. She made a drawing box: a wooden box with a weighted pencil dangling from a string inside and a square of paper lining the bottom. *The City as Written by the City*, a series she has been working on for a decade, is a collection of graphite squiggles documenting walks she has taken in Australia (looking for the house where D.H. Lawrence lived), Florence (clockwise around the Duomo four times) and landscapes much more familiar to me, including a visit to the Toronto Islands, and a walk up Tunnel Mountain with Hamish Fulton during her residency at Alberta's Banff Centre. The images are as abstract as anything I have seen in any gallery, yet that is *my* hometown. Those are *my* mountains. I feel a magnetic pull.

Collier returns and breaks the spell. It's time for us to head to the opening of an exhibition in a town north of Sunderland. "People sometimes come to galleries feeling that they need to understand," he says, "when all they need to do is respond."

When MuchMusic vj Sook-Yin Lee interviewed Radiohead frontman Thom Yorke on the patio behind her house in Toronto, she asked the elusive rock star what or who his god was.

"I don't know," he said. "Not really. He doesn't have a name."

"Do you get a sense of afterlife?"

After saying no, Yorke paused, then corrected himself. "I get it from, like, walking around. The old Wordsworth thing. Walking through the country. You get blown around on a cliff, cowering behind hedgerows in a thunderstorm, things like that."

"Where do you derive solace from?" Lee asked. "What makes you the happiest."

"Swimming in the sea," replied Yorke. "Or walking. Walking, walking, walking, walking. That's fairly normal, isn't it?"

He was quoting his own lyric, from the Radiohead song "Morning Bell." The track might be about divorce, or capitalism, or the suburbs. Or none of the above. The meaning is ambiguous. It's clear, though, that the protagonist yearns for release. "Nobody wants to be a slave," Yorke sings above swelling bass and keyboards and a screaming guitar.

"Walking, walking, walking, walking. Walking, walking, walking, walking. . . ." He is not the only songwriter on this beat.

These boots are made for walking. I walk the line. Take a walk on the wild side. Under the boardwalk. Walking on sunshine. Walk like a man. Walk like an Egyptian. Don't walk away. Walk this way. Walking in Memphis. Walkin' after midnight. Walking on broken glass. I'm walking. Yes, indeed.

In the early 1980s, after taking a freighter across the Pacific to Japan, Art Garfunkel hiked across the island from east to west. He wove through rice fields, using the sun and the horizon as his guides. "The country's not that wide," he said. "The whole thing worked rather well." So one day in 1984, less than 24 hours after making up his mind, he left his apartment in New York wearing a small backpack, cut through Central Park, crossed the George Washington Bridge into New Jersey and kept on going. Over the next 12 years, Garfunkel did three or four legs a year until he reached the coast in Washington State. Most of the time he was alone, with only a map, a notebook and, naturally, a Walkman for company. At first, he would thumb a ride back to the nearest motel room at dusk and, in the morning, return to where he had stopped. Then he switched to "rich man style," and his assistant would fetch him at the end of each day. But there were rules. "Walk Rule No. 1: No peeking. No exceptions," reported *Sports Illustrated*. When getting a ride over unwalked roads, he never looked. "Walk Rule No. 2: Keep moving. Constant starting and stopping is a waste of energy."

"I had my American Express card in my back pocket," Garfunkel said in a radio interview, "but I basically woke up the spirit of travel and replaced that feeling of 'Where's my car keys?' into 'There's west, and I have my map,' and the rest is just follow your sense of direction and cut through the earth as if you were two years old and an unprogrammed human being who is going to just go."

Garfunkel released a live album called *Across America* in 1997. He chose to commemorate the cross-country walk with a collection of oldies, including hits such as the *flâneur* anthem "Feelin' Groovy," which opens with that classic exhortation to slow down (because you're moving too fast). A year later, he flew to Ireland and set out on foot for Istanbul. In the spring of 2014, ready to resume touring after a four-year battle with debilitating vocal-cord weakness, he had reached northern Greece, 370 miles shy of his destination.

Despite decades of anecdotal evidence, there has been very little research into links between creative thought and physical activity. Scientists have deconstructed the mechanics of the human body from head to toe, and the mind is no longer a black box. There is a large literature exploring connections between exercise and various cognitive processes. But we are only starting to understand why and how walking stokes the imagination.

In the first research project of its kind, psychologists from the universities of Kansas and Utah examined the impact of walking in nature on creative problem-solving. Expanding on earlier studies of Attention Restoration Theory, 56 adults involved in Outward Bound wilderness expeditions were sent on four- to six-day hikes in Alaska, Colorado, Washington and Maine. They were cut off from all electronic devices during the experiment. Twenty-four of the study subjects completed a creative reasoning and problem-solving measure called the Remote Associates Test the morning before beginning their backpacking trip; the rest did the test on the morning of day four. The RAT asks participants to come up with a word that can tie together a trio of other words. For instance: cottage, Swiss, cake. The correct response: cheese. Answer 30 to 40 such questions over half an hour, and researchers get a pretty good sense of how fluidly your synapses are firing. The people who did the test near the end of their hikes performed 50 percent better than the control group.

It is difficult to determine to what degree immersion in nature or disconnection from technology is responsible for the difference, the psychologists write in a paper called "Creativity in the Wild." These factors are two sides of the same coin. Most of us live in an environment where the balance between active time in nature and exposure to technology has shifted radically. As immersion in nature declines, there is a reciprocal increase in our use of and dependency on technology. Children now spend an average of around 20 minutes playing outdoors each day in the U.S., and nearly eight hours using a computer, tablet or smartphone or watching TV (and are frequently riveted to more than one device at the same time). All of this digital multitasking and stimulation hijacks our attention and inhibits higher-level cognitive functions. It limits opportunities to benefit from the recuperative qualities of natural environments — the soft fascination at the heart of Attention Restoration Theory.

In a state of soft fascination, the brain is more prone to introspection and mind wandering. This engages its "default mode" network, an interconnected set of regions in the brain that are active during wakeful rest. And this may be important not only for peak psychosocial health, but also for divergent or lateral thinking. Convergent thinking entails following a set of logical steps to reach one solution. Divergent thinking is the non-linear process of exploring many possible solutions.

Geographer Joseph Murphy compared the energy development conflicts in Rossport, Ireland, and Lewis, Scotland, because he saw them while on the same walk. His mobile methodology gave him time to reflect and juxtapose in creative ways. "When you're walking, you encounter things and people which will challenge your worldview, and force you to reorientate," he told me during our hike. "You are allowed less opportunity to remain in your silo, in your existing way of thinking, in your existing way of doing, because you are encountering all the time. Which is not what happens when you get in your car to go somewhere else."

Other than "Creativity in the Wild," the only other quantitative research into walking and creativity I found is being done by Stanford University's Awesomely Adaptive and Advanced Learning and Behavior unit (a.k.a. the AAA Lab). Scientists there conducted a series of experiments using a few different creativity measures, including Guilford's alternate-uses test, which asks subjects to come up with as many possible uses as they can for common household items, and Barron's symbolic equivalence test, which asks people to devise metaphors or "symbolically equivalent images" for a set of phrases (for example, a candle burning down: life ebbing away, water flowing down a drain). Nearly 180 undergraduate psychology students participated. They completed the tests while seated and while walking on a treadmill in a room with blank walls, while walking through Stanford's beautiful California campus and while being pushed through campus in a wheelchair. Their responses were ranked and compared, and the results were clear. Treadmill and outdoor walking increased alternate-uses test scores significantly compared to sitting — walkers came up with an average of around five more alternative uses than sitters — and led to a "residual creativity boost" when subjects were questioned after they had stopped moving. In the Barron's symbolic equivalence test, walkers came up with creative metaphors 95 percent of the time, compared to 50 percent of the time for sitters, with walking outside producing "the most novel and highest quality analogies." And because of the wheelchair test, unlike the wilderness hiking experiment, "the effects of outdoor stimulation and walking were separable."

"I thought walking outside would blow everything out of the water," says AAA Lab educational psychologist Marily Oppezzo, "but walking on a treadmill in a small, boring room still had strong results, which surprised me." I didn't find this to be the case on my tread-desk, though a representative of the manufacturer suggested that had I spent more than a few weeks on the machine, using it would have felt more natural.

Walking does not appear to help people who are immersed in "more focused, convergent types of thinking, such as when you must choose one correct answer," says Oppezzo, who defines creativity as the production of appropriate novelty. She can only speculate about the cognitive responses to walking that stimulate divergent thinking, such as its ability to decrease inhibition, which might prevent us from internally filtering imaginative concepts.

The dual process theory of cognition proposes that we have two main types of thought. System one is autonomous and automatic, fast and emotional; system two is slower, more effortful and logical. Widely accepted by psychologists and popularized by Daniel Kahneman's *Thinking, Fast and Slow*, these dual processes can also explain creativity. The first system helps us make associations between information we already have in memory and information we acquire from the outside world. The second helps us evaluate and refine the ideas formed through the associative process. The result can be a sudden insight, a solution to a problem you have been stuck on — the eureka moment that strikes when you stroll through the park, like James Watt's breakthrough on the steam engine.

When we walk, our senses take in a torrent of new information. These sights, sounds, smells and tactile sensations mingle with past experiences and perceptions. We integrate ideas we might not otherwise put together. This can spark originality, which can come in handy when there are forks in the road.

Creativity is important for a number of reasons, says psychologist Paul Sowden, director of ILLUME: The Faculty Centre for Creativity Research, at the University of Surrey. For individuals, the feeling of having insight, of finding a new way of being in the world, is good for one's sense of purpose and well-being. It helps us face life's challenges. These benefits apply to organizations as well. Creativity can help a company deliver better products or services, and help keep employees satisfied and engaged. It may also help people cope with alcoholism, grief and trauma. Even depression can be seen as a lack of creativity; we can't imagine any possible happy outcomes to our troubles.

"Creativity is fundamental to the human experience," says Sowden. Evolutionarily, it allowed us to adapt to our environment. Today, it "underlies our ability to do things like science or arts. Without understanding creativity and without understanding how we can optimize creativity, both in individuals and in society, we can't optimize our science, our art, our technology, our organizations and, arguably, we can't optimize our individualized living experiences."

Walking can give us time and mental space for creative ideation and evaluation, an incubation period for effortless rumination, for ideas to bubble away. And exercise has been shown to help cognitive flexibility — the ability to think about different concepts at the same time, which can further propel the cross-pollination of ideas. "There are lots of things that creativity relies upon," says Sowden, "and walking will supply them, in one way or another."

While I have him on the phone, I run an idea by Sowden: that there's an ancient bridge between walking and creativity, because both were central to our development as a species. "We have no data that speaks to this," he says. "But we have a correlation. Walking is a strong part of our ancestry, and at some point, the human species became creative."

Sowden suggests I contact one of his occasional collaborators, Liane Gabora, a psychologist at the University of British Columbia's campus in the Okanagan Valley who researches the evolution of creativity. When I awkwardly start to explain my theory, she cuts me off. "Walking and creativity are distinctly connected," says Gabora. "Distinctly connected."

As we began to walk on two legs and stopped using our hands for locomotion, we gained manoeuvrability in our fingers and hands, and we started to think about the kinds of things we could do with these increasingly dexterous digits. We could manipulate objects with precision and modify our environment to a greater extent than any other species. Over thousands of generations, bipedalism and creative thought developed in conjunction with one another.

Anthropologists, archaeologists and psychologists continue to debate the origins and purposes of creativity, just as they still bat around theories of bipedalism. Our earliest known inventions, stone tools most likely used to split fruits and nuts, date back between 2.6 and 1.7 million years. This was the start of an intellectual leap that has given us the ability to send a rocket to the moon, decode DNA and perform breathtaking symphonies. Around 60,000 to 30,000 years ago, our ancestors experienced the "big bang" of creativity. As Gabora writes in a chapter she co-authored for *The Cambridge Handbook of Creativity*, this explosion was marked by the more or less simultaneous appearance of strategic season-specific hunting, elaborate burial rituals, dance, "and many forms of art . . . including naturalistic cave paintings of animals, decorated tools and pottery, bone and antler tools with engraved designs, ivory statues of animals and sea shells, and personal decoration such as beads, pendants, and perforated animal teeth." As our brains continued to grow, Gabora tells me, we gained the ability to encode memories with rich details. After going on a walk, we didn't remember just one massive tree — we could recall the beautiful sky, what the clouds looked like and many different trees. These memories had more roots through which any one recollection could elicit a "reminding event" of another memory. This "recursive recall" allowed us to string memories and abstract thoughts together. We could think about our current physical movements in the context of past movements. We could rehearse and practice skills in our minds. "We could engage in a stream of thoughts," Gabora says, "that could take you from the here and now and into the imagination.

"People get ideas when they are out walking. You are away from things that are demanding your attention. You can stray farther and farther from the present by deconstructing or making sense of what happened in the past, but also by figuring out what could happen in the future."

After a couple million years of evolution, Gabora worries about the impact of contemporary society on creativity. Modern technologies are both increasing and decreasing our capacity for generating novel ideas. New digital tools and a surfeit of free time can inspire us to express ourselves, and to do so in fresh ways. We can reach out and tweet anyone; these conversations can lead *anywhere*. I would not have found Gabora, or read her research, without the internet. But today, the answer to virtually every question is at our fingertips, thanks to Google, and every conceivable physical tool is for sale at

Home Depot (or on Amazon). Moreover, kids spend so much time playing video games, where they *know* there are solutions — they only have to find them — instead of, say, hiking along a creek like the one behind Gabora's house, where there is uncertainty and risk. "It's an unpredictable world, and that's the world humans have always lived in," she says about her creek, "and now we're dealing with virtual worlds that are prefabricated by other human minds, and prefabricated in such a way as to make them addictive. And every other kid out there is confronting exactly the same problem and is forced to come up with exactly the same solution. If they were out there hiking, they would all be encountering slightly different situations and that would be cultivating their minds in slightly different ways, and when they came together they would have a richer, more diverse set of ideas because they faced *different* challenges.

"When you're walking," she continues, "you're seeing the world and hearing the world slightly differently with each step, and that seems conducive to seeing your problems or issues slightly differently as you move forward. This is something people have done for thousands of years. They thought things through as they walked. Just as the terrain looks slightly different the more you move forward, your views and perspective shift slightly."

In the early 1960s, a talented but troubled 19-year-old painter named Ryan Larkin started working for Canada's National Film Board. As a child, Larkin had taken classes at the Montreal School of Fine Arts, where one of his teachers was the Group of Seven's Arthur Lismer. At the NFB, he did animation work on instructional films for the army and navy before catching the eye of legendary director Norman McLaren. Larkin made a couple of successful experimental animated films. In his spare time, while friends went on acid trips and sampled the '60s smorgasbord, he hung out in cafés and bars, watching and sketching people walking around. Larkin lined his small office with mirrors and studied his own form as he walked. He spent two years making the five-minute line drawing and colour wash film "Walking," which weaves together the movements, gestures and expressions of an array of urban characters. Noted for its pioneering style and loosely structured narrative, it was nominated for an Academy Award in 1968 and has been called one of the most important animated films of all time.

I recall watching the film as a kid. It strikes a carefree tone — a solitary figure strides purposefully with hands in his pockets, while people waiting in line for a bus look on jealously — but also has tinges of melancholy and menace. Across artistic genres and geographies, walking symbolism swings wildly between salvation and terror. For every fictional protagonist seeking a new start, there is a book like Cormac McCarthy's *The Road*, a post-apocalyptic journey across a grim land of ash and death. Stephen King evokes the same mood. One of his early novels is *The Long Walk*, about a marathon walking contest in a totalitarian America in which 100 teenage boys must maintain a pace of at least four miles an hour as they walk down the East Coast. Stop walking, you die. The contest ends when there is only one boy left alive.

Walking is also at the heart of King's creative process. After months of writer's block, he came up with the ending to *The Stand* on one of his daily four-mile walks. King was almost killed one afternoon while walking on a two-lane blacktop highway near his summer house in western Maine. A man driving a van was trying to push his Rottweiler's nose out of a cooler full of meat — a detail that sounds like it was lifted from one of King's books — and hit the author head-on. King's left leg was broken in nine places. His right knee was split down the middle. His right hip was fractured. His spine was chipped, four ribs were broken, and the gash in his head required 30 stitches to close. Five operations and two weeks later, he took ten steps in a hospital corridor. Three weeks later, his wife rigged up a desk he could roll to in his wheelchair, and King resumed writing: "I stepped from one word to the next like a very old man finding his way across a stream on a zigzag line of wet stones. . . . There was no miraculous breakthrough that afternoon, unless it was the ordinary miracle that comes with any attempt to create something."

More than anything by King, Ray Bradbury's short story "The Pedestrian" gives me chills. The year is 2053. Leonard Mead loves to walk. Every night, he strolls alone along the buckling concrete sidewalks of an empty, silent city, peering at houses whose residents are riveted to their viewing screens. Suddenly, he is stopped by the city's lone police car. (There is no more crime; nobody goes outside.)

> "Business or profession?" a metallic voice asks.
> "I guess you'd call me a writer."
> "No profession," says the voice. "What are you doing out?"
> "Walking," replies Mead.
> "Walking!"
> "Just walking."
> "Walking, just walking, walking?"
> "Yes, sir."
> "Walking where? For what?"
> "Walking for air. Walking to see."

Mead is told to get into the car. There is no driver. He is taken to the Psychiatric Centre for Research on Regressive Tendencies.

The Dark Mountain Manifesto I told you about in the last chapter is essentially a *cri de coeur* from a group of artists. A passionate reminder to take a look around.

English artist Mike Collier did a 60-mile walk up the River Tyne in 2011 with a quartet of natural historians. Over five summer weekends, with more than 30 members of the public joining in, small groups followed the river from its mouth to the village of Thorneyburn in the hills of Northumberland National Park. Leaving the sea and passing through Newcastle's post-industrial waterfront, where a pedestrian bridge and a contemporary art gallery have replaced coal depots, these rural *flâneurs* encountered an edgeland bursting with life. Interesting things happen in transition zones, where city becomes country, where a riparian habitat becomes a plain, where a forest becomes a field, where day becomes night. When we see a place changing in front of our eyes, we gain insight into our complex, dynamic relationship with the things that it was and the things it may become.

While walking, Collier wrote down the names of all the plants and animals he saw, heard, smelled and touched. After the final weekend, he led a series of workshops in rural communities along the route. Attendees were invited to do short art walks, farm walks and mindfulness walks. Collier made digital copies of 30 pages from his diary and added coloured pastel notations. Displayed in an exhibition called *The Resilience of the Wild*, his field notes explore the nature on our doorstep. Humans have been altering the landscape for centuries, but wildness finds a way to prevail, and we need not travel far to find it.

Collier's art draws the viewer's attention to what exists in the places where he travels. Elastic City's walks encourage you to appreciate what's there, and then to make something new. The collective has branched out geographically from Brooklyn and Manhattan, but its programming generally revolves around the nature in or of a city: an all-night walk along Fire Island, a sliver of land off Long Island that's home to beautiful beaches and a thriving gay scene; a three-day trip to Detroit, which made use of an airplane and a van, but was mostly walking, led by a former Motor City resident who had "some shit to work out" and invited others to join him and do the same.

The Signature Walk is lighter. After making the installation with found objects on the sidewalk, we continue to the intersection of Ocean Avenue and Flatbush. It's about 7:30 p.m., and the rush-hour traffic is finally letting up. A long lineup has formed beside a food-bank truck. Todd Shalom asks us to spend a few minutes studying the text on all the signs within sight, then to compose a poem using only those words. I'm pretty happy with my little verse: "No chicken salad / summer starts with / phat rehab." But Ben Weber, who has a background in theatre, summons his inner beat poet and a deep voice and blows the rest of us away:

Ave flora
Ave Wendy
Ave Flatbush
Shomer Shabbat
No no on the sidewalk
Any size hot
Aqua empire

Something about Weber's performance, probably the way he drops "Shomer Shabbat," makes me realize that despite his all-American name and Wisconsin upbringing, he is Jewish, like Shalom and me. After the walk finishes, with a look at the way the dying light dances across the burnished steel of a phone booth, the three of us discuss our similar secular ways over dinner. Shalom speculates that there might be something very Jewish about Elastic City's walks.

"If you think of Jews historically, they were not allowed to be business owners or property owners," he says. "So what happened? They became accountants, the bankers, the ones who lent the money. But they didn't actually have anything physical. They were the brokers, the ones who were mediating. Perhaps the same thing could be said about an artist leading you on a walk. You're not exactly exchanging something tangible, but you are giving someone an experience."

seven
SPIRIT

"Pilgrimages make it possible to move physically, through the exertions of one's body, step by step, toward those intangible spiritual goals that are otherwise so hard to grasp. We are eternally perplexed by how to move toward forgiveness or healing or truth, but we know how to walk from here to there, however arduous the journey."

— *Rebecca Solnit*, Wanderlust

"If you walk hard enough, you probably don't need any other god."

— *Bruce Chatwin*, In Patagonia

"Would you like a drink to take to your room?"

I have just hiked 21 sun-stroked miles along the cliffs, coves and hedgerow-lined lanes of north Wales, from the small village of Abersoch to the smaller village of Aberdaron, and even though the pub and dining room at the Ship Hotel are overflowing with boisterous fishermen, farmers and English families on holiday, proprietor Alun Harrison can read the look in my eyes. He pulls a pint of ale, cask conditioned at a brewery less than an hour away, and leads me through the Saturday supper-hour hubbub to a room upstairs, where my luggage is waiting. The carpet is slightly shabby and the floor a little slanted, but my window swings open to the crash of waves and the brine of ocean. It's my first day of walking on an ancient pilgrimage route, a land's end where old customs and modern indulgences share the trail. I take a sip and step into the shower. A guy could get used to traditions like this.

I am on the Llŷn Peninsula, the 30-mile-long "arm" of Wales, which reaches west into the Irish Sea just south of the Isle of Anglesey. A travel magazine has asked me to sample a short section of the Wales Coast Path, and to pace out the peninsula's walksheds, the distance one can cover on foot in a day. But in my mind, it's a more lofty mission: a stab at existential clarity in a place where walking is woven into the DNA. A place veined with well-worn paths, heavenly vistas and welcoming villages. A place where the biggest impediment to epiphany might be the local vernacular, which is confounding enough to dislocate your jaw.

The Welsh refer to themselves as Cymry. On the Llŷn — prop- erly pronounced by pushing your tongue against your upper front teeth and making a lispy *clhh* sound (*Clhh-lynn*) — most Cymry speak Cymraeg. Children learn their mother tongue before English at home and school, and the signage is bilingual, which adds to the feeling that you are somewhere truly foreign. Although London is only five hours away, the pace here is much slower and more intimate — a shift akin to the contrast between Ottawa and Atikamekw territory. And in both of these geographically close but culturally distant lands, everybody is *croeso* (welcome) to experience the *hud, hanes a harddwch* (enchantment, history and beauty). This is best done on the Llŷn by *cerdded* (walking). Cymraeg and *cerdded* have endured because of the peninsula's isolation, which has also kept small-scale farming and fishing, and an anachronistic zeal for poetry, very much alive.

My feet are in the hands of outfitter Peter Hewlett, who owns a tour company called the Edge of Wales Walk. He is ferrying my gear from stop to stop. All I have to do is amble along with a light daypack. At least until it's time for the choppy sea crossing.

Pilgrims have been travelling to tiny Bardsey Island, two miles off the tip of the Llŷn, since the early days of Christianity, seeking redemption for their sins. Ynys Enlli is said to be the burial site of

20,000 saints. Three visits equalled one journey to Rome. Today, the ruins of Bardsey's 13th-century Augustinian abbey stand on the site of a 6th-century Celtic monastery. When King Henry VIII cracked down on convents, friaries and other ecclesiastic outposts in the mid-1500s, busting them up and taking their money, the island became a base for pirates and smugglers. Three hundred years later, a small farming and fishing community found purchase.

Sheep and cattle are still raised in the stone-walled pastures of Bardsey, and there are lobster, mackerel and other tasty animals in the surrounding waters. Only a handful of people hunker down in the island's slate-roofed cottages year-round. But the pilgrims, they keep on coming. Over dinner at the Ship, an inn since the 1600s, where I eat crab caught by the owner's brother, Hewlett tells me that some still walk the length of the Llŷn and make the passage to Bardsey for religious reasons. Most of his clients, however, are like me: seeking ecstasy and eternity in a good, long hike.

My route today began beside the harbour in the resort village of Abersoch. The trail climbed through flowering purple heather and yellow gorse to a single track that clings to the edge of the Cilan headland. Every field was fenced, but Wales Coast Path insignias bade me through gates and over stiles, and onto private land. Sheep grazed lazily, kestrels hovered in the offshore breeze and sailboats bobbed in the blue down below. Stopping to rest in a field of rye, watching the golden blades ripple in the wind, I felt it, already — that swelling of body, mind and spirit. Also, stirring in my muscles, rolling through my stomach, tingling my temples and throat, there was something else . . . something more visceral. Thirst.

At home, I usually walk with enough water to douse a campfire, and food to last a fortnight. Maybe the luxury of the luggage shuttle made me lightheaded, but I had brought less than a litre to drink, and a couple packets of cookies pinched from hotel rooms. After five hours under the hot sun, I rebooted with a swim at sprawling Hell's Mouth beach, and filled my bottle in the washroom of an

Elizabethan estate now run as a museum, nabbing an apple from a tree in the garden before leaving. Descending into the postcard visage of Aberdaron, a cluster of whitewashed buildings above a sandy beach, green hills stretching to the horizon, the forbidden-fruit symbolism made me smile.

The next morning, encouraged by Hewlett, hungover, I go to church.

St. Hywyn's, a double-naved stone-and-timber structure originally built nearly 1,000 years ago on the bones of a Celtic oratory, is across the street from the Ship, just above the pounding surf. "It's nice," says Rev. Susan Blagden, looking out over the congregation, augmented this Sunday by vacationers, "that we're able to welcome occasional churchgoers." I sit in the rear pews, shielded by a young couple with a baby, and scan a history pamphlet as Blagden leads the prayers. St. Hywyn's has served as a sanctuary for centuries. Like the Hebrew cities of refuge, it offered fugitives an opportunity to sit tight and reach an understanding with their adversaries. This came in handy if your adversary was a malicious tribal chieftain. It also helps rebuff more insidious threats.

Blagden has just returned to the Llŷn from attending a retreat, and her sermon today is about the need to declutter our busy lives. "What power does your smartphone have?" she asks. "Only the power that you give it." My ears perk up; I put down the pamphlet. "In today's Western culture, we find it very difficult to know what's enough." Of course, it's not always possible to go away on retreat, she adds, advising parishioners to take time each day to be still in their heads and hearts.

"Amen," I whisper, offering the affirmation without irony for the first time in my life.

One of Blagden's predecessors at St. Hywyn's, Vicar R.S. Thomas, the second most famous poet with this surname in Wales, was a notoriously Spartan man. He believed that local peasants were simple folk, and thus the closest people on earth to god. His canon was no *Child's Christmas in Wales.* "The rain and wind are hard masters," R.S. wrote in one of his poems, "Too Late." "I have known you to wince under their lash."

I sneak away from church when the mother slips outside with her crying baby. Within seconds, it starts to rain.

Today's hike takes me around Llŷn's end and back to Aberdaron, and I don't mind getting wet, knowing there's another ale-and-shower combo at the end of the trail. My first stop is St. Mary's Well, a sacred spring that pilgrims have been drinking out of for hundreds of years, their last blessing before the perilous rowboat trip to Bardsey. I shuffle down a slippery, natural-stone staircase deep into a jagged cleft and follow a narrow black-rock catwalk to the mossy, triangular pool. Perched above the roiling tide — suspended, as D.S. wrote, between sea and sky — I cup my hands and take a few sips of the cool, sweet water, then head back up into the mist.

Some people ooze inner calm. They know themselves. They may not have figured out the meaning of life, but they have puzzled together a decent understanding of their own lives. Even if it's an act, I'm jealous. That convergent feeling I get while walking — it seldom lasts long.

Most of us are a little lost and confused, at least some of the time. Which is why, when not preoccupied with basic needs, when drifting and drooling off to sleep, or daydreaming at the desk, we wonder. We worry. We yearn. For *something*. Humans are uniquely curious creatures. An evolutionary quirk called neoteny left us with juvenile characteristics well into maturity. Unlike other mammals, we remain inquisitive as adults. And so when the stars line up, when opportunity arises, we grant ourselves a sabbatical — an hour, a long weekend, an open ticket — and heed the elemental urge to go stumbling down the trapline of the soul.

A pilgrimage is a journey to a special place. *Journey, special, place*: these words are entirely subjective. Whether sacred or secular, it is a quest for salvation, inspiration, guidance or some combination thereof. An outward effort to balance our inner lives. Muslims go to

Mecca. Hindus bathe in the Ganges. Jews push prayers into cracks in Jerusalem's Wailing Wall. A Vietnam War veteran might press his palm against the black granite memorial in Washington, D.C. A baseball fanatic buys the *Field of Dreams* audiobook and takes a road trip to the Hall of Fame in Cooperstown, N.Y. Stanley Vollant leads communal expeditions from reserve to reserve. I hoof it to the family cottage. Or try to, anyway.

With all those unoccupied hours to ruminate, we look inward while wayfaring, and we don't always recognize what — or who — we see. Anthropologists Edith and Victor Turner believe pilgrims are in a liminal state, between past and future identities, awash in possibility. There is a symbiosis between journey and arrival, writes Rebecca Solnit, and a "delicate line between the spiritual and the material." We cross a threshold into an ethereal geography and, awed by the enormity of our questions, proceed the same way our ancestors explored. With two feet and a heartbeat.

Buddhist monks can attain enlightenment through walking meditation. They pace back and forth on paths no more than 30 to 60 feet long, sometimes for a full day. The two ends provide a structure, and sharpen awareness. The physical activity engages and relaxes the mind at the same time, providing the energy to focus on every step. If you manage to apply such mindfulness to daily life, former Buddhist monk John Cianciosi writes in *Yoga Journal*, your consciousness will remain alert and alive, "transforming ordinary life into a continuous practice of meditation, and transforming the mundane into the spiritual." Having "nothing else to do and nowhere to go," he adds, "can be truly liberating."

Few of us are this disciplined. We follow the crowd.

El Camino de Santiago, one of the oldest continuously walked pilgrimages on the planet, is actually a web of trails. On a map, they resemble tributaries flowing into the main branch of a river. The 500-mile Camino Francés, the route completed by Vollant (and by the grieving father played by Martin Sheen in *The Way*), is the most popular. Starting in St. Jean Pied-de-Port, France, it crosses the

Pyrenees into Spain and, shadowing Roman trade tracks, heads west through farmland, forest, mountains, village and cities, on or near paved roads roughly half of the time.

Francis Tapon, a globetrotting Californian who has walked across the United States four times and trekked throughout Africa, Central America and Europe, calls the Camino the most overrated long-distance trail on earth. "About 95 percent of the time, car traffic is within earshot," he wrote after completing the journey. "With endless bars, restaurants, hotels, vending machines, tour groups, you're hardly removed from the 'real world.'" While Tapon admires the mental toughness required to finish the Camino, his criticisms are widely lambasted by commenters for whom the walk was life-altering.

After about a month on the trail, pilgrims pass through the doors of the cathedral in Santiago de Compostela, where the bones of St. James the Great, one of the 12 apostles of Jesus, were "discovered" in 813 AD. Some continue an additional 60 miles to the tip of Cape Finisterre, an important edge of the world to ancient Celts. Like the journey to Bardsey, the Camino appropriates the paths of those who came before.

The Codex Calixtinus, an illustrated 12th-century manuscript put together by a French friar, offered advice on reaching Santiago. Europe's first guidebook sent flocks of walkers across Spain. Millions attempted the Camino in the Middle Ages — the largest movement of people in Europe at the time. It was a convenient destination, easier to reach than Jerusalem, and for some, depending on their starting point, more attainable than Rome. Medieval wars and plagues interrupted the flow, as have modern conflicts. But despite the erosion of Christian piety in much of the Western world, numbers have been climbing in recent years, spurred by cheap travel, and by the publication of books such as Paulo Coelho's *The Pilgrimage* in 1987 — the novel that spoke to Vollant from his bedside table. (British travel writer Tim Moore's account of doing the walk with a donkey might not have inspired hordes of copycats, but actor Shirley MacLaine's Camino memoir surely tilted the ratio of New Agers to

Catholics toward the crystal set.) More than 215,000 people made it to the shrine of St. James in 2013, three times as many as a decade earlier.

Roughly 3 million people do the Hajj in Mecca each year. Every able-bodied Muslim is supposed to visit the holy Saudi Arabian city at least once in their lifetime. It is an act of Islamic solidarity, and submission to god. Most take planes, trains and automobiles to get there (a few trek thousands of miles on foot), but the heart of the ritual consists of walking seven counterclockwise laps around the Kaaba, the cuboid building at the centre of the Al-Masjid al-Haram mosque. Photographs invariably show an ocean of people clad in simple white garments, regardless of their wealth or status. The circumambulation represents oneness and unity, each lap a different phase of our lives, and replicates the natural order of the universe: planets circling the sun, electrons around a nucleus.

Mecca's attendance is eclipsed by the Kumbh Mela, a Hindu dip in a sacred river, which rotates between four locations in northern India. The 2013 pilgrimage, at Allahabad, where the waters of the Ganges, Yamuna and Saraswati meet, drew more than 100 million people. Roughly 30 million people bathed on a single day, the largest gathering anywhere on the planet — ever. A tent city forms during the Kumbh Mela. At night, the temperature can fall to just above freezing. Waste disposal and sanitation facilities are rudimentary. Diseases such as cholera and meningitis spread. The noise, around 85 decibels on an average day, is loud enough to cause hearing damage. Three dozen people died in a stampede at Allahabad's train station in 2013, a regular risk, even in years when a mere 10 million people show up.

From the outside, the atmosphere at the Kumbh Mela sounds dangerous or, at a minimum, stressful. Twenty thousand people were separated from their friends and relatives on the day of the world's biggest baptism. It can take three hours to push a mile through the crowds. Yet pilgrims typically depart feeling serene and blissful, according to Stephen Reicher, a psychologist at the University of St. Andrews in Scotland, who led a six-year research project on the Kumbh Mela. Participants develop a shared identity and report smoother and more rewarding social relations than Hindus who stayed home.

Though it's the opposite of meditation, congregating generally makes people feel good. We experience mutual trust, respect and cooperation. Support from others helps us become more resilient. In spite of the conditions at the Kumbh Mela, pilgrims reported improved physical health after it finished. Mind over matter may be a factor, but Reicher's research also demonstrates "the power of collective experience in transforming everyday life," he wrote in a dispatch for the *Guardian*. "It shows how a sense of shared identity provides the underpinning for that sense of community and civility about which so much is spoken."

Compared to the crush of the Kumbh Mela and the Hajj, the Camino is a walk in the clouds. It may not remove you from the world of billboards, electricity transmission towers and industrial parks, but proximity to cities and towns, and an ample network of *albergues* and *refugios* with cheap meals and beds, eliminate the need to carry a heavy load. They also provide youth hostel–style camaraderie, if you can handle the dorm-room snoring. You might fall into friendly conversation, share a meal, maybe form a pack with convivial strangers — or take off on your own, depending on the rhythm you feel. Unless you're seeking a solo path to enlightenment, these amenities are a big draw. It's a lot harder to thru-hike the Appalachian Trail, or to walk across America.

"In this space you can achieve a direct human interaction that doesn't take into account hierarchies, so people become intimate very quickly," Ellen Badone, an anthropology and religious studies professor at McMaster University, writes about the Camino in her book *Intersecting Journeys: The Anthropology of Pilgrimage and Tourism*. "Stepping into this extraordinary sphere leads to extraordinary interactions."

Gideon Lewis-Kraus decided to do the Camino while on a drunken bender in Estonia. The friend he was visiting, American author Tom Bissell, was researching the tombs of the 12 apostles, and Lewis-Kraus (a restless writer in his late 20s who had moved from San Francisco to freewheeling Berlin in a preemptive strike against future regret) agreed to tag along. At overnight stops and on the trail in the Pyrenees, the pair hang out with and informally interview dozens of pilgrims, most of them young and from Europe or North America. Few are motivated by religion. Few, including Lewis-Kraus, the son of two rabbis, can articulate why they are walking. Still, the experience was moving enough to send him on a deeper journey.

In *A Sense of Direction: Pilgrimage for the Restless and the Hopeful*, Lewis-Kraus writes about crossing Spain, his ensuing 750-mile circular walk between 88 Buddhist temples on the Japanese island of Shikoku, and a visit to the Ukrainian city of Uman with his brother and father during the annual Rosh Hashanah pilgrimage to the grave of a Hassidic mystic. The book, philosophical treatise meets travelogue, captures the joy and pain of the Camino and the colder, lonelier Shikoku circuit, and provides a forum for Lewis-Kraus to probe his troubled relationship with his father, who came out of the closet in his mid-40s and abandoned the family to make up for lost years. All of this is funnelled into a meditation on the nature of the pilgrimage.

Academic literature views these journeys as "ritual experiences that represent breaks from the ordered configuration of everyday life," writes Lewis-Kraus. "The pilgrim could step outside of *all* roles and just *be a person*, someone without responsibilities or expectations or constraints besides continuous forward movement to a distant goal." Cynics see the contemporary Camino as a cheap backpacking jaunt, but he argues that the appeal is "ritual continuity," that the mode of travel itself matters. If the divine model is sin, penance and redemption, the corresponding lay path leads from anxiety to austerity to forgiveness. In the end, although he and Bissell and their travel mates cry and hug in an emotional daze upon entering the cathedral in Santiago de Compostela, Lewis-Kraus is left with a question: "Five hundred miles, and now what?"

Some pilgrims never stop. On New Year's Day, 1953, 44-year-old Mildred Ryder set out on foot for New York from Pasadena, California. The U.S. was mired in the Korean War, the Cold War and McCarthyism. Ryder, who wore a blue tunic with "Peace Pilgrim" written in white capital letters on the front, wanted to rouse people from apathy. "Humanity, with fearful, faltering steps, walks a knife-edge between abysmal chaos and a new renaissance, while strong forces push toward chaos," she wrote. "Yet there is hope."

A series of revelations had initiated Ryder's metamorphosis into the Peace Pilgrim. After growing up poor and outside the church on her parents' poultry farm in New Jersey, she took secretarial jobs and married a businessman. In 1938, discomfited by her relative prosperity during the Great Depression, she went for an all-night walk in the woods and prayed for guidance. A profound peace came over her. She would dedicate her life to giving, not getting.

Ryder's husband was drafted into the army after the attack on Pearl Harbor, and she refused to accompany him to training camp. They drifted farther apart when he was overseas and soon divorced. She simplified her life by reducing her wardrobe to two dresses, forsaking meat and embarking on wilderness treks. In 1952, Ryder became the first woman to hike the entire Appalachian Trail in one season. On a hill overlooking rural New England, she had a vision: "I saw a map of the United States with the large cities marked — and it was as though someone had taken a colored crayon and marked a zigzag line across, coast to coast and border to border. . . . I knew what I was to do. I will talk to everyone who will listen to me about the way to peace."

Ryder departed Pasadena penniless. She planned to fast until given food, and not to stop until given shelter. Over the next 28 years, the slender, five-foot-two woman with white hair crisscrossed the country seven times, migrating north in summer and south in winter, venturing into Canada and Mexico. When nobody offered her a bed, she slept in fields and under bridges, in drainage pipes and beside the road, in cemeteries and New York's Grand Central Station.

She gave presentations in community centres, churches, schools and private homes, introducing herself during these talks and to strangers beside the highway as a pilgrim "walking not *to a place* but *for an idea*," writes biographer Marta Daniels. "Her definition of peace included peace among nations, among people and individuals, and the most important peace — within oneself — for only with inner peace, she believed, can the other kinds be achieved." Ryder said that people needed two things to lead a meaningful life: a calling or "path of service"; and something, religion or art or nature, that would "awaken their higher nature."

The Peace Pilgrim stopped counting her miles at 25,000 in 1964. By Daniels' estimate — 29 pairs of sneakers averaging 1,500 miles per pair — she had covered 43,500 miles by 1981. That year, in demand as a speaker and increasingly accepting drives to reach events on time, a car she was riding in was hit head-on by another vehicle outside Knox, Indiana. She died just after impact.

Mildred Ryder's peripatetic proselytizing was ahead of its time. She foreshadowed a shift from pilgrimage as an appeal for divine intervention to pilgrimage as a demand for political change, writes Solnit. Although she came after Gandhi, she predated the civil-rights era and the birth of charity walkathons, and the continued fusion of personal marathons with protest marches, all calls for a world not as it is but as it should be.

We can't all stride ceaselessly toward harmony. Even people on epic pilgrimages usually have a goal line. In his mid-40s, confronting a mid-life crisis, Jean Béliveau — a Montrealer but not the hockey legend — closed his neon-sign business and packed a three-wheeled running stroller with food, clothing, a tent and a sleeping bag. On August 18, 2000, he kissed his wife and grown children and left the city for an around-the-world walk dedicated to raising awareness about the violence afflicting children throughout the planet. (Sounds fanciful, but the first decade of the 2000s was the United Nations' International Decade for a Culture of Peace and Non-violence for the Children of the World. Also, his wife flew to meet up with him from time to time.)

Béliveau came close to quitting in Ethiopia, had an emergency prostate operation in Algeria, met Nelson Mandela and three other Nobel Peace Prize laureates, and absorbed lessons from the peasants he spent time with in impoverished countries such as Peru and Mozambique. "They have a sustainable way of life," he told one interviewer. "Who are we to teach them? We are destroying our planet, putting so much stress on our society. It's time to learn from them."

Do not follow my footsteps, Béliveau said upon returning to Montreal, 11 years and 46,000 miles later. Make your own.

Paul Salopek is on a journalistic pilgrimage. In 2013, the *National Geographic* writer started a seven-year, 21,000-mile walk from Ethiopia to Tierra del Fuego, "retracing on foot the global migration of our ancestors." His Out of Eden project aims to address the major stories of the Anthropocene, from climate change to technological evolution and cultural survival. Among his first stops were the West Bank (during the Israeli attack on Gaza) and the divided island of Cyprus. A two-time Pulitzer Prize winner and a veteran foreign correspondent, he has come to believe that parachuting into a war zone to cover a conflict limits your perspective. Instead, by "inching slowly across the surface of the earth," he hopes to discover "links between stories . . . that are covered in a really granular, segmented way by the media.

"Maybe the most important thing that people might find extreme," says Salopek, "is the capacity to wait, which the global north seems to find increasingly incomprehensible. The ability to sit under a tree and wait for something to happen — it's a way of perceiving the world that is getting rarer as the world becomes more wired."

Salopek acknowledges that he may not last seven years on the road, that he might have to abandon the walk at some point. Pilgrimages don't always work out as planned. You can get sick, or injured, or assaulted. Or realize you are heading in the wrong direction.

For every Jean Béliveau, there are dozens of Daryl Watsons. The young American playwright was desperate for a "mission statement." A devout Christian as a teenager, he had left the Church. For a year, he wrestled with fear and doubt, dreaming fitfully every night about his purpose on earth. So in 2009, he adopted a new name, Peace Pilgrim, and departed Delaware on a six-month walk to San Francisco, in search of a renewed connection to god.

Like his namesake, Watson shed his possessions. He sealed all of his money inside an envelope, wrote "For Charity" on it and dropped the cash into a mailbox. "Why aren't more people giving away everything that they own and walking across the country?" he says in an episode of NPR's *This American Life*, rationalizing his impulsive decision. "When you live in this world, as crazy as it is, *this* is what you do."

On the first night of his journey, Watson slept on the cold concrete outside a Catholic church; on night two, in the dugout of a college-town baseball diamond, wrapped up in a piece of Astroturf. Three days after beginning, cold and tired and sore and hungry, he gave up. Watson sobbed his story to the night manager of a highway-side Best Western, then phoned his mother, who paid for a room. Sitting in a hot bath, he realized that the paralyzing questions that had been tormenting him were no longer urgent. "Being so exhausted . . . I didn't care anymore if I had the answer," he says. "It just wasn't important."

I have more in common with the new Peace Pilgrim than the original one. My eyes are bigger than my guts. That aborted walk to the cottage, remember, was not without precedent.

At dawn on my 35th birthday, while living in Edmonton, I stepped off our front porch into an August thunderstorm to attempt a seven-day circumnavigation of the 200-mile Waskahegan Trail. The loop traverses parkland, boreal forest and, thanks to handshake deals with landowners, private meadows and pastures. It follows marshy lake-shores and grassy river valleys, and intersects the occasional town. More mundane than majestic, it's a flat swath of central Alberta that thousands of people drive through daily. But to me, at the time, with twin toddlers at home and a start-up magazine to pilot at the office, it sounded like paradise: a childless, cheap and safe adventure.

(That last criteria was crucial. If I got badly hurt doing something so ill-conceived, Lisa would have killed me.)

It took me three hours to reach the city's southern boundary. At an on-ramp for the main highway to Calgary, I stuck out my thumb. A cabbie named Gall picked me up and drove me 10 miles to a range road that led to the first official trailhead. "You should do the West Coast Trail instead," he said, describing his bear and cougar encounters in the Pacific Rim rainforest. "*That's* wilderness."

Yet once I turned off the pavement and started walking along the shore of one of those sloughy, skinny bodies of water that prairie folk call a lake, I saw pelicans flapping in formation overhead and ducks erupting from the water's edge. A grey heron begrudgingly took flight. Hawks shrieked. Deer darted. A pileated woodpecker pecked. Windmilling through nettles above my head and stutter-stepping over cow shit, I stopped to smell the sage and ate the season's last raspberries.

That night, after hiking more than 30 miles, I stayed with a farm family whose land the trail passes through. Lloyd Schnick plucked me from his neighbour's barley field — we had talked on the phone a few days earlier; he said to drop by — and his wife, Charlene, served up a meal of chicken with beets, potatoes and peas from their garden. She showed me to a spare room in the basement, put my soaked clothes in the dryer and, in the morning, after a bacon-and-egg breakfast, slipped me a baggie of peanut butter cookies. The Schnicks accompanied me down to the lake at the foot of their property and waved goodbye from a point jutting out into the water as I climbed over a stile onto the next farmer's land.

Buoyed by their generosity, I was in that liminal state described by Edith and Victor Turner. I felt kinship, connection — and, soon, pain. Within an hour, my right knee began to hurt. Bad. My back and shoulders, bearing a needlessly hefty pack (*two* novels? two *hardcover* novels?), were not doing much better. The deadfall on the path from a recent tornado was nearly impenetrable, and my aging boots were waterlogged. By noon, I was popping ibuprofen. At 3 p.m., I discovered I had made a mathematical error: Camrose, the small city where I had intended to overnight, was still 25 miles away.

What's the point of pushing on, I asked myself, if I'm miserable? I thought back to something one of the trail's founders had told me when I pried him for route details: "Sure, you could do the whole thing in one go, but I prefer to take my time and, well, *enjoy* it."

Defeated, I called Lisa and asked for a ride home. And though I completed the Waskahegan in stages over the next three months, any lessons I learned were soon forgotten.

Mapping out the route to my parents' cottage, I budgeted four days for 114 miles. I pictured myself strolling in the resplendent autumn leaves, chewing a sprig of straw, napping under the canopies of oaks and elms. In addition to this delusion, I made other mistakes: too much gear, too much food, too-new boots. By day two, wrong turns had notched up the mileage, and my blisters had blisters. I stubbornly ate my squished peanut butter sandwiches while passing farm stands and chip trucks. There were traces of bliss — whenever I *stopped* walking. For instance, during the two boat rides I had arranged in advance. An 84-year-old marina owner motored me across Balsam Lake after I joined him and the staff for coffee and tall tales in their scuttlebutt shed. Early the next morning, a teenaged lodge handyman took me up the misty Gull River into the town of Minden, where I disembarked on the public dock beside the downtown bridge and began the final stretch.

Limping north, sliding toward my decision to surrender, I realized I had again planned to go too far, too fast. Regardless of the metaphysical potential of a journey, it's difficult to meditate on the meaning of anything if you are fixated on counting miles and the looming darkness.

Ultimately, it was Lisa, meeting me at the cottage with our daughters, who supplied a saving grace: she had brought my slippers, the only footwear my pulpy feet could handle.

George Mallory tried to reach the top of Mount Everest because it was there. He was fixated on the summit — and died on his third attempt.

The Camino, or the far shore of a vast country, or any long-distance, soul-seeking journey, holds a similar attraction. It is *there*. I am *here*. Something will be revealed along the way. *Solvitur ambulando*.

In his book *The Road Is How: A Prairie Pilgrimage Through Nature, Desire and Soul*, naturalist Trevor Herriot chronicles a pilgrimage of modest distance but ambitious scope. He sets out from his house in Regina on a 40-mile, three-day hike to the land east of the city where his family has a small cabin and a large garden. Much of Herriot's writing explores the rich layers of life that endure in the cropped-over grasslands and riverine coulees that the rest of us tend to neglect, eyes drawn to the bold mountains farther west or the oceans that bookend the nation. This walk is a return to familiar terrain, the subtle wildness in his native Saskatchewan, only now, in his early 50s, Herriot's focus is internal. Recovering from a bone-breaking misstep off a ladder, cranky about the destruction of nature and community at the hands of profit-hungry government and corporate minders, he wants to discover what's wrong with himself: "It was as though my years as the know-it-all naturalist had rendered me deaf to the very spirits that might be able to help me grow up or heal or whatever it is I am supposed to do at this stage of life."

It could be a manifestation of my own obsessions with walking and environmental Armageddon, but pilgrimage lit appears to be trending. When things get tough, the lost go looking. Mourning and heartbroken, Cheryl Strayed found herself on the Pacific Crest Trail in the bestseller *Wild*. Milquetoast Harold Fry, British novelist Rachel Joyce's unlikely protagonist, left his home in England and, instead of mailing a letter to a deathly ill friend, personally delivered it to her bedside, more than 600 miles away (a fictional trek echoing film-maker Werner Herzog's walk from Munich to Paris to visit the ailing critic Lotte Eisner). Mirroring the early 20th-century American poet Vachel Lindsay, who traded poetry for food and lodging on several inter-state hikes (Illinois to New Mexico, New York to Ohio), British poet Simon Armitage hiked the 268-mile Pennine Way, exchanging nightly readings for beer and bed and breakfast. "In many ways," he writes in *Walking Home*, "the Pennine Way is a pointless exercise, leading from nowhere in particular to nowhere in particular, via no particular route, for no particular reason. But to embark on the walk is to surrender to its lore and to submit to its logic, and to take up a challenge against the self."

Herriot roots around for metaphor and meaning in the ditches and pastures that line the route to his cabin, gazing up at the constellations as his sandals sink into the mud at the bottom of a slough. He finds symbiotic beauty in biological processes, in the microscopic minutiae of pollination, in the networking capabilities of mycorrhizal fungi. Before beginning his walk, Herriot camped on a hill by himself and fasted, as directed by an Aboriginal friend. After three days and three nights of "boredom and misery punctuated by moments of dread and anxiety," a question had arisen: how does one stop "wandering around in mid-life adolescence . . . how do I finally grow up in my relationships?" And he knew where to look for answers. Friends of his had travelled to Nepal and Machu Picchu, but he wondered whether we can "separate spirituality from bodily life and culture, both of which are profoundly connected to soil, climate, and the other givens of place. . . .

"If it's good to eat locally," asks Herriot, "isn't it just as good to heal and feed our souls locally?"

I finish reading Herriot's book on a grey spring morning in Ottawa. For weeks, I have been deskbound, absorbed by adventures in Spain and other far-flung locales. I lace up my hiking boots. There is a greenbelt around the corner from my house, a string of parks and marshes that might eventually be bulldozed into a road. It is a weekday, and I see only one dog walker when I pass through a thicket of willows and sit on a picnic table on a low ridge, serenaded by twittering redwinged blackbirds in courtship. There's that feeling again.

I cross the busy street that borders the green space and enter a low-income townhouse and apartment community called Heron Gate Village. The sidewalks abound with women wearing colourful burkas and mothers pushing babies in the strollers, unlike the deserted white Pleasantville of my own residential enclave. Behind and between the towers and low-rises, I find a lattice of wooded paths linking the curvy roads to the area's parks, schools and shopping strips. It is five minutes by foot from my house, and I have never been on these walkways before.

Like Herriot, I am steered in a proximal direction. My sights, I have come to understand, are set next door. I'm more interested in Matt Green's daily walks in New York than his cross-country trek. I'm not infatuated with one summit. I walk because *something* is *everywhere*. Every day can be a pilgrimage, if the goal is a deeper sense of your small role in the revolving world.

Forgiveness and healing may be elusive targets, but honesty is still within range. Walking exposes us to the immediate physical reality. And though our brains distort and deceive, though we have more confidence than competence, though self-delusion steers us toward flattering conclusions, when we walk, our thoughts become more clear as the body and mind align. Pace and mood modulate into cadence. Observations and ideas merge and furnish our best bet at truth. Or, as the Welsh say, *gwirionedd*.

On the Llŷn, after I drink from St. Mary's Well, I'm on another vertiginous single track. The 500-foot granite cliffs on the eastern flank of Bardsey Island rise from the sea to my left. Today's route hugs the rim of the peninsula's headland, then cuts across its neck back to Aberdaron. An easy 13-mile loop. I have enough water and food. My boots are worked in and waterproof. My rain gear keeps me dry. Bleating sheep keep me company. The wildflowers and craggy shoreline look stunning. Yet each step feels heavy, ponderous. It's not a physical weariness or discomfort. It's a nagging sensation. I have been away from home for two weeks now. It is a holiday weekend in Canada. I'm not sure what Lisa and the girls are doing, only that I am not with them, and that summer is slipping away. Christians and their Celtic forebears may find answers on this path, but maybe I should be looking closer to home.

It is still raining the next morning. Rob Jones, who works for the Welsh national tourism bureau, meets me in the Ship's dining room for breakfast. We're supposed to travel to Bardsey together, but a hard wind is blowing. The boatman has advised us to check with him in a couple hours.

We hop into Thomas's car and drive up the hill from the hotel to outfitter Peter Hewlett's house for tea. On the wall of his den hangs a colourful poster titled "The Broad and Narrow Way," originally made in Germany around 1850. Conveying an evangelical Christian perspective, the illustration depicts the two paths we all must choose between: virtuous living or worldly pleasure. The narrow route on the right side of the poster leads past green trees and shrubs and Christ on the cross to a mountain that is surrounded by winged angels and bathed in golden light. The wide road on the left is lined by a ballroom, a gambling hall, a tavern and "Sunday trains." Dotted with men whipping donkeys and fighting, it culminates at a dark castle where panicked stick figures are consumed by flames. Named and numbered verses from the Bible are scattered throughout. "Dan 5:27" is in the top-left corner, just above the fires of hell. Hewlett takes a Bible off his bookshelf and finds the verse with my name: "Thou art weighed in the balances, and art found wanting."

Thomas and I still have some time on our hands, so we visit Felin Uchaf, an educational centre devoted to breathing new life into traditional Welsh skills. Three miles from Aberdaron, on what was once a bare, windswept parcel of land, volunteers have planted thousands of trees and bountiful organic gardens, and fashioned eco-friendly buildings using local stone, earth, thatch and timber. Among the workshops taught at the centre are sessions on straw-bale construction, earth and cob walling, thatching and timber framing. Volunteers come from around the world. As they learn, the facility grows. There is an energy-efficient barn, a boat-building shed and several medieval-style roundhouses. Water reeds cut from nearby marshes are used for roofing. Sheep's wool is batted together and put into the walls for insulation.

Dafydd Davies-Hughes, the soft-spoken project manager with a beatific smile, leads Thomas and me into a roundhouse, whose base is dug into the earth. Its design is styled after an Iron Age meeting house. There are benches and bunks built into the mud walls and a hearth in the middle. In addition to providing accommodation for workers, students and travellers, Felin Uchaf hosts storytelling events, fireside gatherings where performers enthrall audiences with nothing more than their voice. "People come to the Llŷn on a pilgrimage, seeking something, but not everybody makes it to Bardsey," says Davies-Hughes, an accomplished storyteller himself, but also a renaissance man with experience as a biologist, teacher, farmer and builder. "So this is a stopping place, to celebrate all of the cultures that have passed through here, the churning of stories that is Europe. It is still a frontier. The elements you meet here — the wind, the rain, the sun — they're very strong, compared to the warmer valleys inland. People like the rawness of that. Everything is tamed now in our world.

"There's an archetype here," he continues, speaking more broadly about the Llŷn, just as Rory Stewart read the Lune as more than a river. "There's a stretching out to the west. People have long looked at this journey as an echo of what human beings go through in their lives. They pass though the mainland and come out on this little pinnacle of land. The water that separates us from Bardsey, people see it as the Sea of Forgetfulness, or the River Styx. A stepping stone to heaven. The peninsula is a route toward that. It's a meeting place, a threshold, the edge of the known world. Though it might be symbolic, you come to the edge of a life, and what goes on beyond here is unknown."

Thomas's cellphone rings. Our ship sails in 15 minutes.

Porth Meudwy — Port of the Hermits, in English — is the only place to launch a boat on the turbulent coastline beyond Aberdaron. A muddy road descends through a deep cleft in the cliffs to a narrow rocky beach with a cracked concrete slipway. Skipper Colin Evans tells us to climb into his bright yellow 30-foot catamaran, which sits on land atop a trailer that is hooked up to a tractor. "I'm sorry, lads, it's a bit wet today," he shouts above the roaring wind. "I'd like you to wear lifejackets."

With a fuzzy brown beard and massive forearms, Evans looks like the type of person only a fool would ignore, even on a calm day. He is wearing a yellow rain slicker over a blue sweater, and a pair of bibbed grey-green rubberized fishing pants rise to his chest. Another man sits at the wheel of the tractor and reverses into the surf, which lifts the boat off the trailer. Evans has made this crossing around 10,000 times, completing his first solo sailing at age 16. He guns the throttle. We pull away from the inlet and start bucking wildly in the waves.

"This is only half as bad as it gets," Evans tells me as the boat pitches up and over swells, spray crashing onto the deck, "and we'll travel in twice as bad as this — if we have to." Storms and fierce currents in these waters have claimed more than 70 ships. In 2000, a gale stranded 17 visitors on the island for two weeks.

We round the cliffs that I saw during my walk yesterday, and the sea flattens. A red-and-white lighthouse presides over Bardsey's patchwork of green fields. Owned and managed by a charitable trust, about a mile and a half long from north to south and half a mile wide, the island is a national nature reserve, a sanctuary for migratory birds and rare plants. This makes it a destination not only for the devout, and hikers, but also for scientists, who come to Bardsey's bird observatory to do research on species such as the Manx shearwater, a daredevil flyer that can live more than 50 years. Only 2,000 day visitors are allowed each year. "But it's still a working island," Evans says. There are about 370 sheep and a couple dozen cows and bulls. "It's not just about conservation. Well, it is, really, in a way. It's about the conservation of an old way of life."

Evans's family has been farming and fishing here since at least the 1700s, maybe longer. His father worked the lobster traps and was a lighthouse keeper. His mother is an acclaimed poet. Colin, too, has a way with words. "This crossing," he says, "represents the continuation of an old tradition. My whole life is built around perpetuating old traditions, because they're sustainable. They represent a way forward. The past is the future."

We putter toward the beach at the southern end of Bardsey, where another tractor pulls us onto land. This harbour is protected from the prevailing winds. It's a better landing place than any other port in the area, which means that sailors have always kept their boats on the island, not the mainland, and that the seafaring skills have stayed here too.

Evans wonders whether there will be anything to keep his children on Bardsey when they grow up. There are possibilities: crab processing, sausage making, fish smoking, kayak tours. But the island has had a "wobbly" few decades; economic development has stalled. Still, he says, it feels natural to balance farming and fishing with conservation, research and tourism. Because there are families with a historical attachment to the island, there are people here to care for it.

The Celtic and Christian pilgrimages to Bardsey are a relatively recent phenomenon, Evans says, now in tour-guide mode. Mesolithic flint found on the island indicates that it was inhabited 5,000 to 10,000 years ago. There is also evidence of Bronze Age cremation sites. There was a spiritual pull long before any church.

Thomas and I walk away from the water on a rutted dirt road, inspecting the ruins of the abbey and peeking over stone walls at the cottages available for summer rental. We enter the tiny chapel, and he sits at the organ and plays. I give Thomas a nod and leave him to his hymn.

I wander around alone for a couple of hours. Although 20 people live on the island in the summer, and there are a couple dozen scientists and visitors here today, Evans's words during the crossing prove prophetic: Bardsey has a mysterious ability to swallow people. I don't see another soul.

As I climb a sheep trail to the island's highpoint, the sun re-emerges for the first time in two days. Travelling the length of the Llŷn was once a journey of penance. Now, I realize, it is simply a way to get perspective on the rest of the world.

"The mountain conveniently hides the mainland, as though it was placed there on purpose," Evans had told me down below. "You can forget about the mainland when you're here, and you might do. In bad weather, you might as well be 1,000 miles away.

"I think that this island fosters independent thought. It's close — but far. The hubbub of life is just a little while away, but you might not be able to get to it. That makes you feel different. The only thing you can see is a distant goal."

eight
FAMILY

"Let children walk with nature, let them see the beautiful blendings and communions of death and life, their joyous inseparable unity, as taught in woods and meadows, plains and mountains and streams of our blessed star."

— *John Muir*, A Thousand-Mile Walk to the Gulf

"We're so marinated in the culture of speed that we almost fail to notice the toll it takes on every aspect of our lives. Sometimes it takes a wake-up call to alert us to the fact that we're hurrying through our lives instead of actually living them."

— *Carl Honoré*, In Praise of Slow

The car drove over my legs just above the ankle.

Maggie got hit first. She was on her bike. I was jogging behind her. Daisy trailed a couple pedal strokes back. We were four blocks from home on a bright, crisp morning in mid-September, the ash and maple leaves already tipped with crimson. After dropping off my daughters at school, I planned to go for a run along the river, then sit down to work.

We had a green light and were between the white lines of a pedestrian crossing. Maggie was halfway through the intersection when a car coming from the opposite direction turned right, head-on into our path.

"Stop!" I yelled. To Maggie, to the driver.

Then: the sickening sound of metal and plastic crunching together.

Maggie fell into my chest and we tumbled backwards onto the road. Her pink-and-grey bike disappeared beneath the bumper. Flat on the pavement, I arched my neck in time to watch the passenger-side front tire of a compact suv roll over my shins. Shock and adrenalin muted the pain.

Two thoughts flashed through my mind when I saw the car on my legs. First: there's a car on my legs. Then: Maggie!

I looked left. She was sitting on the street beside me. Not screaming. Not crying. Not bleeding. *Intact.* I looked right. Daisy stood over her bike, holding the handlebars tightly, more curious than concerned.

The corner jammed with rush-hour commuters. Vehicles backed up in all four directions. A man with a phone at his ear said an ambulance was on the way. Within seconds, a woman was crouching beside Maggie. "I'm a doctor," she said. "Show me where it hurts?" Maggie pointed to a small cut on her left knee, the only visible wound.

"Oh my god! Oh my god!" shrieked the suv's driver, hands cupped in front of her mouth. "Are you okay? Are you okay? Are you . . ."

"Could somebody please get her away from us," I said, swept by a need to maintain calm for the girls. A bystander ushered away the driver.

Less than a minute later, a police officer pulled up. She recruited the man with the phone and they helped me stand and hobble to a strip of grass between the street and the sidewalk. I lay down again, nauseous. A pair of paramedics removed my mangled shoes and cut off my socks. They examined my lower body without alarm, then lifted me onto a stretcher. Maggie climbed into the back of the ambulance on her own. A friend who happened to be passing by escorted Daisy the rest of the way to school. My shins began to burn as we drove away, but we had been incredibly lucky.

The police officer came to the hospital to take our statement. The driver, she told us, had just dropped off her son at the school.

Lisa arrived in time to watch a wisecracking emergency-room physician dig a pebble out of the gash in my right ankle. Frequent sessions with the vacuum cleaner, he insisted while stitching me up, would be the most effective form of rehab. Then he looked at the x-rays, confirmed that no bones were broken and said, "Let's get you on your feet."

Most mornings, my daughters and I walk to their school. It is half a mile from our house. Twelve hundred and fifty footsteps. It is often my favourite 15 minutes of the day.

There are no sidewalks the first three blocks, wide residential streets with little traffic. Maggie and Daisy rescue worms from the road after spring rains and, in winter, balance atop plow-packed ridges of snow. We scan the treetops for cardinals and crows, or kick skittering pucks of ice. The girls pepper me with questions: about the rainbow of signs that sprout during election campaigns, about the rocks and minerals embedded in the asphalt, about bullies and bragging, and the utility of homework. I answer with tangents and wordplay. Maggie and Daisy roll their eyes at my dad jokes, then unleash their own stream-of-consciousness humour. I tell them stories about my childhood, and they reciprocate with revelations about emotions and encounters heretofore shrouded by youthful secrecy or the distracting cornucopia of all that transpires in a day. When they're not sparring with words or fists, or words about each other's fists, or attempting to sing pop songs louder than one another, the girls speak to each other with familial tenderness. Fraternal twins, removed from the territorial battles of home, travelling together through a confusing world. Our conversations flutter like butterflies, bobbing unpredictably along a boundless path.

The best time to talk to your kids, says author and food activist Michael Pollan, is when you are making a meal together. Side by side at the kitchen counter, chopping, stirring, there is no eye contact. Even a teenager will let down his or her guard. Walking shuffles you into the same parallel alignment. Alongside a friend or relative, or even a casual acquaintance, your footfalls can settle into an unconscious synchronicity — an indicator of social interaction, say cognitive neuroscientists at Caltech. This type of movement synchrony, a pair of Dutch psychologists write in a 2011 paper, can be a sign of "shared feelings of rapport, an affective state of mutual attention and positivity." Simultaneously soothed and stimulated by the motion, you are primed to open up, and to listen to what someone else has to say. An intimacy develops — between lovers or siblings or pals, or between parent and child, but also a maturation of the relationship between you and your surroundings. A mindful immersion in the realm within which you exist. A grounding in *your* world.

Walking is like dancing, says author and slow-living advocate Carl Honoré: two or more bodies moving at the same tempo, cooperating and communicating, forging a tacit partnership. "Away from clocks and technology and the distractions of the modern world, walking creates a vast, open space for things to happen, and that's often when relationships flower and blossom most," he tells me. "We are physical beings. So much of how we express ourselves and how we interact with the world and with other people is bodily, it's corporal. If you find a shared rhythm with someone, that opens up another level of intellectual and emotional flow and exchange."

To Honoré, walking is also a simple, free and accessible first step toward overcoming the "virus of hurry" that is coursing through our veins. A habit that compels us to count minutes instead of savouring them; to do everything as quickly as we can, not as well as possible. A habit that can inhibit the growth of healthy, reciprocal relationships. "Walking turns you inward, toward that internal monologue which is such an important part of being human, of living the examined life," says Honoré. "But it also opens you up to the textures and details of the world around you — and to other people. These are two sides of the same coin. After turning inward, you have more to give when you turn back out to the person who is walking with you. There's more of you in play."

My trips to school with Maggie and Daisy are not always idyllic. The girls can be best friends, or pathological rivals. But even when they bicker and try my patience, even when I'm stressed or in a rush and ready to trigger an argument, we're in a shared flux, figuring out how to relate. And whatever our moods, we're deepening the bond between our little unit and the community we live in. Every parent knows how easy it is to dig in your heels when embroiled in an infantile debate — no, *you* started it! — but on our morning walks, we are pulled from these skirmishes by office-bound neighbours who greet us by name, and by retirees who wave from living-room picture windows. And then we join the stream of children and parents that swells as it nears the school, trickles of meltwater replenishing a river during the spring freshet. Our salutations and conversations may seem trivial, but they are a glue. A reminder of our mutual stake in a daily ritual.

Maggie and Daisy, who were eight when the accident occurred, still jockey to hold my hands, though goodbye hugs on school grounds are considered embarrassing by Grade 4. The cliché holds: they grow up fast. Soon the girls will hit puberty. The social and cultural dynamics they must navigate are already complex, and changing quickly. They will inherit a world vastly different from mine. If walking can help us find a common tempo, maybe it can also soften this transition. For them, and for me.

There is only one busy corner to traverse on our commute, the intersection of Alta Vista Drive and Randall Avenue. We pass through it twice a day, five days a week, 10 months of the year. The quadrant closest to our house is kitty-corner from the schoolyard. Unless it is clogged with traffic, cars zip along Alta Vista, a house-lined, two-lane thoroughfare with a speed limit of just above 30 miles per hour. Drivers sometimes turn off and onto Randall, the street that fronts the school, without looking carefully for pedestrians or cyclists. But for the most part, it is an ordinary and orderly semi-suburban corner. Until it isn't.

Forty years ago, when I was toddler, around two-thirds of North American children and teenagers walked or cycled to school. Today, despite the fact that so many of us now live in cities, roughly one-third make the trip under their own steam. In the U.S., 89 percent of students from kindergarten to Grade 8 who lived within one mile of their school in 1969 walked or cycled; today, 35 percent cover that short distance on foot or by bike. In Canada, a 2012 report pegged the number of kids shuttled to school in personal vehicles at 41 percent, up from 13 percent when their parents were young. (Perhaps more foreboding, more than three-quarters of children between the ages of three and five can use a computer mouse, but less than half know their own address.)

In its 2014 report card, a non-profit called Active Healthy Kids Canada gave the country's children a D- on overall physical activity — the same score as the U.S., Ireland and Australia, but a lower rank than Colombia, Ghana, Mexico, Mozambique, Nigeria and five other nations. Only Scotland, with an F, fared worse. Although 84 percent of Canadian three- and four-year-olds meet minimum activity guidelines, just 7 percent of kids aged five to 11 manage an hour of daily activity, a figure that falls to 4 percent among teenagers. "Our country values efficiency — doing more in less time — which may be at direct odds with promoting children's health," the report card declares. "We have engineered opportunities for spontaneous movement (such as getting to places on foot and playing outdoors) out of our kids' daily lives."

Urban planners, municipal politicians, medical doctors, psychologists, epidemiologists and environmentalists have started to zero in on the walk to school. Surgeons circling around a patient, preparing to operate. It is a regular bout of exercise in an era of epidemic obesity and diabetes, they tell us. It can curb anxiety and spark mental acuity. It treads lightly on the planet. It cuts traffic congestion and makes streets safer and more vibrant, encouraging others to take to their feet. It gives children time with their parents and, as they get older, an opportunity for graduated independence in an overprotective, over-programmed world. And it can help counterbalance a toxic culture of "harried parenting and rampant materialism," argues British psychotherapist Graham Music, that is making kids meaner and more self-absorbed. "Children with low empathy," he says, "are turning into narcissistic adults who have never learned the intrinsic rewards of social belonging and interdependence." The ability to share and understand somebody else's feelings, Australian philosopher Roman Krznaric writes in *Empathy: A Handbook for Revolution*, "has the power to transform relationships, from the personal to the political, and create fundamental social change."

Kids who travel predominantly on foot or by bike perceive their neighbourhoods differently than those who are chauffeured around in a car. American urban design researcher Bruce Appleyard asked nine- and ten-year-olds from two similar suburban pockets outside Oakland, California, to draw "cognitive maps" of the routes between their homes and schools. They were instructed to indicate places they liked or disliked, dangerous locations, the houses of friends and other spots where they hung out. In Parkmead, with its heavy traffic and minimal active transit, the children "frequently expressed feelings of dislike and danger and were unable to represent any detail of the surrounding environment," Appleyard writes. In Gregory Gardens, which was similar to Parkmead, but with about half the traffic and markedly slower vehicular speeds, the children's maps showed "a much richer sense of their environment" — more houses, trees and places to play, and fewer dangers and dislikes. Walking to school gave kids a more holistic appreciation of their neighbourhood.

Appleyard appears destined to do this type of research. His father, humanist urban designer Donald Appleyard, wrote the seminal book *Livable Streets*. It empirically demonstrated that people who live on city streets with lighter traffic have more friends and acquaintances than those who live on streets with heavy traffic, and that as traffic volumes increase, the space that people consider to be "their territory" shrinks. This possessive feeling translates into a sense of connectedness, because there is more "exchange space" in which to interact. Or, as Dan Burden of the Walkable and Livable Communities Institute says, "Cars are happiest when there are no other cars around. People are happiest when there are other people around."

Before she became the City of Toronto's chief planner, Jennifer Keesmaat gained a following around a TED Talk she gave on the importance of walking to school. She discusses physical health and our collective carbon bonfire, and the value of local, daily responses to both crises. The walk to school is also a rite of passage, says Keesmaat, recalling her 1.7-mile journey as a child. The rain, the jackets that were too thin, the shoes that got soaked, the paper lunch bags that got wet and then ripped apart, forcing her to figure out how to get runaway apples to her locker. Walking to school cultivates childhood autonomy, she says, which helps create autonomous adults: "It is a simple, hopeful, powerful act. It is an indicator of the health of our children, the health of our environment, the health of our communities."

Walking is not sexy, Keesmaat says to me when we meet in her office on the 12th floor of City Hall. It doesn't dominate news cycles like Toronto's crack-smoking then-mayor Rob Ford, who was being hounded by the dozens of reporters I had to squeeze past on my way to the elevator. Still, she emphatically declares that walking is at the heart of her strategy to transform the city. When Keesmaat discusses this subject with colleagues, there is a usually a strange moment, she says, when people realize that focusing on this "essential part of everyday life is actually a radical idea."

We stopped walking to school for many reasons. Fear of strangers. Fear of cars. Neighbourhoods and streets built for vehicles, not pedestrians. Larger schools located farther from the homes of students, often on the edges of new communities where land is cheaper. Schools being sited and designed without transportation plans in mind. Specialized pedagogical programming on the other side of town. Mostly, though, it's time and convenience. No matter what our days hold, we're generally in a rush. Drive the kids to school, drive to work, pick up the dry-cleaning, pick up the kids, get takeout, get to gymnastics practice and piano lessons and the tutor's house. And repeat. "Busyness has acquired social status," Brigid Schulte writes in *Overwhelmed: Work, Love, and Play When No One Has the Time,* and "keeping up with the Joneses now means trying to outschedule them."

The themes that run through this book — physical and mental health, social cohesion, economic and environmental sustainability, political sincerity, creative and spiritual fulfillment — can all be considered through the prism of the walk to school. It is a fulcrum. A line in the sand. In the urban West, where our wired, globalized lives instantaneously connect us not only to the other side of the city, but also to the other side of the planet, walking to school can serve as one of the foundations of a re-engagement with our own families, and with the people and places that populate our neighbourhoods. It is a way to reintegrate physical and human geography, and help renew a dwindling culture of empathy.

My grandmother lives in a 15th-floor condominium in the northeastern Toronto neighbourhood of Don Mills, Canada's first master-planned suburb when it was developed in the 1950s. Its layout — curving roads and cul-de-sacs, strip malls and ribbons of green space — was used as a blueprint across the country. Pedestrian routes were included in the design, but cars quickly took over. From my grandmother's balcony, I can see the spot where speedway-like Don Mills Road splits into separate northbound and southbound channels. In between lies Peanut Plaza, so named for its hourglass shape. The central island is home to shops, a community centre, a church and a pair of schools. Students must cross three lanes of traffic to get to class.

The area around Peanut Plaza was one of the locations assessed in the report on the walkability of Toronto's high-rise neighbourhoods that I mentioned in Chapter 3. Only one-third of residents feel it's a good place to be a pedestrian. Footpaths linking the dead ends and twisting streets were part of the original plan, but some have been blocked by fences over the years. People make their own shortcuts. Chain link is peeled aside; dirt paths are blazed across grass. But these desire lines lack lighting, snow clearance and other upkeep — a serious threat to safety, say the majority of survey respondents. Moreover, streets such as Don Mills have narrow sidewalks that directly abut fast-moving traffic. There are few crosswalks, and signal times are often too short to permit safe passage. "Although these roads were conceived as facilities for moving vehicles as efficiently as possible," the report says, "they now act as de facto local main streets for high-rise residents and must be traversed to access most destinations."

A few years ago, on her way home, my grandmother warily eyed a pair of teenagers on the far sidewalk as she crossed Don Mills. She was still in the middle of the road as the light turned and traffic started racing toward her. The teens took her arms and helped her hustle over the curb.

The obstacles that make it difficult or dangerous to walk in a city disproportionately affect its most vulnerable residents: children, the elderly, people with disabilities or limited means. As I witnessed in Glasgow, walking helps ward off isolation and depression, in addition to all the physical benefits. As the population ages in Europe and North America, a built environment and programs that encourage mobility among seniors will become increasingly critical. Walking, says Dr. Michael Pratt of the Centers for Disease Control and Prevention in Atlanta, "can mean the difference between a continual fulfilled life or the beginning of their demise."

The Peanut's pedestrian shortcomings don't concern my grandmother anymore. She doesn't get out much. Now in her mid-90s, she has been living on her own since my grandfather died in 2007. The makeup of her building reflects the United Nations mix of the area. Friends from China, Iran and Jamaica keep an eye on her. They bring her dishes from home. When it's not too cold or too hot, she will take a taxi to the nearby supermarket, then walk the two long downhill blocks back to her condo. She brings her "Cadillac," a walker with a padded seat and a mesh basket, and keeps an emergency stash of painkillers and chocolate in her fanny pack. Although my parents and her neighbours constantly offer to pick up whatever she might need, Grandma is reluctant to say yes. A solo excursion to the supermarket is a badge of independence.

I accompanied her on a recent trip. As we strolled the aisles side by side, me pushing the cart, Grandma driving the Caddy, a sack of flour here, a bunch of bananas there, she continued the story that had started at her kitchen table. A story she has been telling me for years. The walk that saved her life, and begat mine.

Tyla was 19 years old and living in southeastern Poland when the Nazi bombardment began. German soldiers overran her village. In December 1939, after her father was beaten and hauled away because he was Jewish, Tyla and her friend David set out from Staszów for the Russian border. For five days, pretending to be brother and sister, they walked east. Peasants gave them potatoes and borscht and let them sleep in their chicken coops. They hid in ditches whenever they saw soldiers. "It didn't kill me doing it," Grandma said, suspiciously inspecting the best-before date on a carton of soy milk, "so it won't kill me talking about it."

At the border, they were stopped by Russian troops while crossing an icy stream and were forced to wait in no man's land. Eventually, they were allowed to enter and registered for factory jobs in the Urals, the Soviet's northern industrial backbone. Thrown together with people from a multitude of faiths, they were worried only about survival, not synagogue. In the spring of 1941, no longer just friends, they went south to work in what is now the republic of Georgia. While growing up, my grandfather had loved walking in the forests around Staszów. During the war, it was a necessity: to get to the factory, to scrounge for food or medicine. In June 1941, the Nazis attacked Russia and he was conscripted. My mother was born that fall.

After the war, her family returned to Poland, then followed relatives to New York, landing in Brooklyn, in that apartment across the street from Prospect Park. Despite a couple of muggings, and long hours on the production line at a shoe factory, my grandfather rediscovered the joy of walking. A ravine path, a routine errand — it didn't matter. Years later, even a trip to Peanut Plaza carried the scent of freedom.

I rarely walked when I was a child. As soon as I could balance on two legs, my mother likes to say, I ran. Yet my parents persisted. They dragged my two brothers and me on weekend hikes along the Niagara Escarpment west of Toronto. When I wasn't racing ahead over a tangle of roots or jumping over chasms between the rocks, I would whine that I was tired and hungry, a refrain I also deployed in the city during forced marches to distant restaurants. We had no television at home until I was a teenager, and this was considered a healthy evening's entertainment. My mother did not drive, so outings with her (to the library, to movies, to the mall) invariably involved a walk, if only to the bus stop. She cajoled us onward with cookies and calmness, but it was the normalcy with which she treated the act — how else are we going to get there? — that instilled an affinity.

As much as I complained, something fundamental happened during those walks. I gained a comfort with the natural world, and a sense of my own stamina. I began to grasp the scale of our neighbourhood and how it fit into the wider urban picture. I shared observations and theories with my parents, and they had time to listen and debate. And my two brothers and I bonded. With no friends or comic books or hockey cards to distract us, we negotiated ways to amuse and tolerate each other.

When I was seven, I started walking two-thirds of a mile to school without adult supervision, forming a pack with friends along the way. I can still draw a map to the monster homes that replaced the bungalows where my classmates used to live. Along with the weekend hikes and restaurant expeditions, those trips laid new grooves atop inherited memories of war and exile. The seed took.

First the dogs chased us. Then we were shocked by an electric fence. And then the undergrowth gave me a rash.

Lisa and I have gone on some epic treks together. We've seen thundering bison in the prairies, the sun rising above a range of snow-capped volcanoes in Alaska, whales spouting under a full moon in the Bay of Fundy. We have taken lazy Sunday-afternoon strolls to our favourite diner, on the other side of the river, for pie. Those were the early days of coupledom. Before mortgages and parenthood, before bad knees and failing eyesight. Holding hands, silent or speaking, our stories began to twine. But often it took a misadventure, like the time we got lost in the Pyrenees, after the menacing hounds and the electrocution, to prompt a new chapter.

We were on holiday in a small town in Spain and had been at a club until 4 a.m. the night before, but I was determined to stick to our plan (read: *my* plan). Hitchhike to the picturesque medieval hamlet at the end of a zigzagging mountain road. Walk a dozen or so dreamy miles through forests and farms. Back in time for a shower at the hotel before dinner.

Our slow start got us to the trailhead at noon. Six hours and several wrong turns later, we had covered barely one-quarter of the route. Boots soaked from repeated river crossings, food and water gone, no sign of any path, I suggested we climb the peak we had just unintentionally circled. "Maybe," I said cheerfully, to compensate for my many blunders, "we'll be able to see the road."

Two things about the way I walk have consistently annoyed Lisa in the two decades that we have been together: I always look for shortcuts, and I seldom agree to stop until I know what's around the bend. This is not a great combination when you are lost.

Walking with your partner is usually good for a relationship. It gives you time to focus on one another, to figure out what's important. "You feel like a twosome . . . you're talking as a team," Howard Scott writes in the *Boston Globe*. "There's a subtle strengthening of the spousal bond." Even if that bond is threatening to snap.

Hiking mishaps have managed to reinforce the elasticity of the union between Lisa and me. When I misread a map and mix up miles and kilometres, or neglect to notice the contour lines, the extra distance or elevation can lead to tension. Yet we always make it home. Over the years, I have been learning to choose our routes collaboratively, to modulate my impulse to press on, and to listen when Lisa says that the rocky ledge where we are is as good a place as any for a picnic. I don't always heed. I need to be reminded that the quality of our mileage matters more than its quantity. But in the Pyrenees, exhausted, defeated, I realized, finally, though not for the last time, that our hike was not about my speed, stamina or superior route-finding skills. It was, simply, about *us*. It was time to climb until we could see the road, make a beeline for it and flag down a ride.

These days, when Lisa and I have an evening to ourselves, our dates often begin with a walk. Even if we're in the green space around the corner from our house, the experience can be transcendent. An orange sunset reflecting off the concrete-and-glass towers of Heron Gate Village, the sweet scent of Japanese lilac on the wind. We talk as we walk. About our aging parents, our aging children, and our aging selves. About trails left behind, and places we will go. About those big fears — environmental apocalypse, economic collapse, runaway technology — and how they don't seem so bad right here, right now. About finding that fine line between the Broad and Narrow ways. By the time we emerge from the woods, our worries have receded.

My daughters and I remained skittish at the corner of Alta Vista and Randall for months after the accident. Maggie was nervous whenever we rode our bikes to school. It was *our* corner, yet every time a car turned a little too tight, or braked a little late, my heart would race. I glared at offending drivers, and purposefully slowed while crossing. There are children here, I thought self-righteously. Slow down.

One winter morning, alone, as I was on my way home, a car skidded to a stop in the same spot where we were hit, its bumper about four feet from my legs. I approached the driver's window. A woman slid down the glass.

"I have the right of way here," I said slowly, shaking.

"I'm sorry," she replied. "I didn't see you."

"There's a school right there," I said, pointing over my shoulder. "Children cross here."

"I'm sorry. I didn't see you. I'm sorry. What would you like me to say?"

"Don't be sorry. Just look. Please. Next time, look."

Back at my computer, I did what any self-respecting, soft-handed city dweller would do. I sent an angry email to my municipal councillor. And, emboldened by indignation, I copied anybody else who might care: the school principal, the parent council, walking advocacy groups. My daughters will be in Grade 5 next year, I wrote, and they should be able to walk to school on their own. What can the city do to make this intersection safer? Traffic calming? Better signage? A crossing guard? Do we have to wait until a child is seriously injured before something is done?

A week later, I was on the phone with one of the councillor's assistants. Changes are coming to that corner, she promised. The painted white lines demarking the crosswalks were scheduled to be replaced by "high-visibility crossings," in this case textured brick surfaces. Such crossings are more noticeable to motorists, who are then more inclined to cede the right-of-way to pedestrians, say traffic researchers. One experiment, in San Francisco, involving the comparison of treated and control intersections, determined that 37 percent fewer vehicle-pedestrian accidents occurred at crossings with high-visibility surfaces or markings. Another study, in Clearwater, Florida, found that drivers yielded to foot traffic up to 40 percent more when crossings were made more visible.

What's more, I was told by the councillor's office, the City of Ottawa's Public Works Department would conduct a traffic count at Alta Vista and Randall to determine whether additional safety measures were warranted. One option was a leading pedestrian interval phase signal, which gives pedestrians an exclusive advance green light for about five seconds, allowing them to start crossing and make themselves more noticeable before drivers start moving. LPI signals, says the New York–based National Association of City Transportation Officials, can reduce pedestrian-vehicle collisions by 60 percent.

I was thrilled. My elected representative at work!

Then I received the results of the traffic count. In two-hour windows around the morning and afternoon school bells, 112 and 119 pedestrians had been counted, respectively — not enough to justify additional interventions. The city's traffic operations technician did note, however, that several adults neglected to press the button that activates the walking-man icon, so "information / guidance sign Mx-38" would be installed to "remind pedestrians of the proper procedures they should follow when crossing the street."

Disappointed, I did something I swore would never happen. I attended a parent council meeting.

As I sat in the school library with a dozen women, my concerns joined a chorus. Parents frequently pull dangerous U-turns on Randall, the principal said. A teacher's car had recently been hit. Drivers ignore the crossing guards. They speed, and park in no-stopping zones, obstructing sightlines and walking paths. Whenever the police or bylaw officers are called, they never arrive quickly enough to ticket offenders. "What are we teaching our children?" one mother asked. "Is this how we want them to behave?"

Eleven adults are standing in a circle in the foyer of Queen Elizabeth Public School on a mild May morning. The squat brick building is on a fast-moving commercial artery in the blue-collar east end of Ottawa. Nearly 350 students, from junior kindergarten to Grade 8, attend. Forty-seven percent live in what the province deems "lower-income" households, and 40 percent have a first language other than English. Socio-economic and cultural barriers limit the number of children who walk or cycle to school, especially in the colder months, says Queen Elizabeth's principal. Still, Kateri Deschenes wanted to increase the number of students who use active transit, and to make the school zone safer for those who already do. So she started talking to Wallace Beaton, the man who convened today's gathering.

Beaton is the regional coordinator of the national School Travel Planning project. Over the past eight months, he and STP's Jessica Sheridan have conducted surveys to determine how Queen

Elizabeth's students get to school, polled teachers and parents about travel habits and observed traffic patterns and spots that are dangerous to pedestrians and cyclists on and around school property. Today, Sheridan is leading a walkabout to inspect these locations, and then a discussion about how best to address all of the obstacles, real and perceived. And she is joined by people who can actually implement changes: a police officer, a bylaw officer, the City of Ottawa's school traffic safety coordinator, two representatives from the city's transit company, a public health nurse, a teacher, a parent and the principal. It takes a village, in 2014, to get a child to walk to school.

Our first stop is the semicircular driveway in front of the main doors. There are no lines on the asphalt indicating where to park, nor any stop signs where exiting vehicles intersect the sidewalk. Double-parked cars are a hazard for children, Sheridan says, reading a list of complaints from a clipboard. Then she points to a single rusted bicycle rack, tucked away by the side doors. A prominent, shiny rack can entice more kids onto two wheels. Positive peer pressure. The STP "stakeholders" nod and take notes. Normally, I detest the s-word. But in this case, whether by altering the architecture, enforcing the law or mounting awareness and educational campaigns, the stakeholders are keeping aloft the same tent.

We follow Sheridan to the edge of the school property and, at a set of lights, cross busy St. Laurent Boulevard. The pedestrian signal here is short, she says, which leaves kids stranded on the median and prompts some to jaywalk. There's a bus stop on the far side of St. Laurent, and the first after-school bus arrives at 3:40 p.m., just 10 minutes after classes finish. This makes students rush and jaywalk despite the heavy traffic.

"The next bus comes in 15 minutes," says one of the transit company reps.

"When you're in Grade 6," counters Beaton, "15 minutes feels like a lifetime."

We proceed to another half-dozen problem spots, where Sheridan recites complaints: illegal U-turns, faded zebra stripes at crosswalks, absentee sidewalks, cars accelerating above 50 miles an hour. Back at the school, in a small meeting room, the group discusses each location and what can be done. Beaton promises to get in touch with his contacts at the school board about painting and signage in the drop-off zone, including anti-idling signs. The transit rep says he will look into pushing back the 3:40 p.m. bus. Ottawa's school traffic safety coordinator will try to get the city's signals group to lengthen the crossing duration and reduce the response time when people push the pedestrian button on St. Laurent, changes that can be implemented within specific windows around the school bell. The city can also set up radar-activated speed boards on St. Laurent. These not only show drivers how fast they are travelling — and scare some into slowing down — but also record data that is shared with the police force. Enough evidence of speeding can spur additional enforcement. A traffic cop can be assigned to watch and hammer bad drivers with tickets, says the police officer.

"Here's what I know about people," he adds. "Ninety percent of the time, they don't pay attention and they lack common sense. But a few tickets tend to alter behaviour."

University of Toronto pediatric orthopaedic surgeon and traffic injury researcher Andrew Howard is trying to determine which school-zone safety measures might be most effective. He led a 2012 literature review of 85 walking and child pedestrian injury studies. All were conducted in highly motorized regions (Australia, Japan, New Zealand, North America and Western Europe), and all met a strict set of criteria (nearly 13,000 articles were considered initially). Among kids in Canada aged five to nine, pedestrian collisions are tied with car accidents as the leading cause of unintentional-injury death. Roughly 55 child pedestrians are killed and 780 are hospitalized with serious injuries every year. These rates fell 50 percent between 1994 and 2003, a trend in other countries as well. But that's because children don't walk as much as they used to, a decline "most apparent for school trips." When kids do walk to school, accidents happen. "Almost 50 percent of all child pedestrian collisions occurred during school transportation times . . . the highest density of collisions occurred within 150 metres of a school." Across the 85 studies, the review concluded, "only traffic calming and the presence of playgrounds / recreation areas were consistently associated with more walking and less pedestrian injury."

Another paper, published by Howard and his colleagues in 2014, explored whether increased walking to school would lead to a rise in child pedestrian collisions. Nine years of Toronto Police Service school-zone accident statistics for children aged four to 12 were analyzed, and travel behaviour was observed at dozens of the city's elementary schools. There were many variables differentiating the neighbourhoods: multi-family dwelling density; traffic light, traffic calming and one-way street density; school crossing-guard presence; and socio-economic status. Ultimately, the paper states, it is not the proportion of people walking but the urban form that has a bigger impact on pedestrian collisions. Road-design features have the closest relationship to accident rates. Mostly, the places where we cross the street. The paths that link where we are to just about everywhere else.

As the conversation continues around Queen Elizabeth's boardroom table, I start to understand how difficult it can be to implement even a single new safety measure. For a child, the walk to school is one seamless journey. It doesn't matter whether they are on city, school board or private property. But responsibility for their safe passage is shouldered by a spectrum of parties, some of which have been prioritizing cars for a very long time.

Beaton got involved with the STP project's parent organization, a non-profit called Green Communities Canada, as a volunteer. He used to make a living working on big-picture environmental issues for NGOs, but it often felt like the *Titanic* was bearing down on him. He hit a wall. He needed to concentrate on smaller changes. Active travel had been eroding for decades, Beaton realized, wearing a reflective sash in the parking lot of his daughters' school. Late-night, side-of-the-desk advocacy work by parents has a low ceiling. Today, STP is his full-time job. In Ottawa, the program is funded by the city's school transportation authority, which operates the school bus net-work. Ontario's education ministry spends about $860 million a year on school transportation, the vast majority of which goes toward busing, a service that carries around a third of the province's students. This cost has spiked from roughly $600 million a dozen years ago. Every child has a right to be bused if they live beyond a certain distance from their school. But a sliver of this budget could accomplish a great deal if allocated toward promoting and supporting active transit, says Beaton. "We're not talking big dollars. You can do a lot with some policy, some bodies and very little money."

The built environment can be prohibitively expensive to retrofit. A decision we make every morning is easier to tweak. If you can, start walking to school once a week, Beaton advises. Walk part of the way. Or simply lay off the gas and let a kid cross the street. The earth-moving can follow. "We've created a school transit culture — stressed parents blasting through stop signs — that is about meeting *our* needs, our adult time pressures. Ask any teacher: they know the students who walked or biked to school. They are energized, they're awake, they're ready to learn."

Sheridan and Beaton are devising an action plan for Queen Elizabeth PS and will spend a full year working with the principal, her staff and parents to implement it. Twenty schools in Ottawa have participated in the STP program since its inception in 2010. Hopefully my daughters' school will be one of the next to sign on; I attended another parent council meeting to lobby for a commitment. At some schools, the success has been phenomenal: the number of students walking and cycling at one school near downtown Ottawa more than doubled from 27 to 65 percent. In the U.S., a national Safe Routes to School centre was established in 2006. Between 2007 and 2012, the number of schools participating in STP-like programs jumped from 1,833 to 13,863, in all 50 states, and rates of walking to and from school increased from 12.4 to 15.7 percent in the morning, and 15.8 to 19.7 percent in the afternoon, with the biggest growth occurring at low-income schools. Kateri Deschenes does not know how significantly the numbers will change at Queen Elizabeth. But as she tells me after the stakeholders disperse, all of this effort will at least introduce a new mindset to some students: "I *can* walk. And I might do so in the future."

Ontario's Highway 401 is the busiest freeway in North America. Some days, more than 500,000 vehicles drive a 14-lane segment that cuts through Toronto. My grandmother's balcony faces the highway from the north. The house where I grew up is a dozen blocks to the south. July, rush hour on a Monday morning, I am on the highway, heading west, against the current, away from the city. Maggie and Daisy are with me. The school year is over. We're going hiking.

Our destination is the Bruce Trail, the longest and oldest marked footpath in Canada. The route, now 550 miles, officially opened in 1967, the country's centennial year. Founder Ray Lowes envisioned a strip of land that would be left alone, not manicured or developed. "It's not too much to ask," he said. "A later generation will demand it." The trail follows the Niagara Escarpment away from the American border, bisecting Hamilton and skirting the fringe of the Greater Toronto Area on the way to its northern terminus, a cairn at the tip of the Bruce Peninsula.

Since Maggie and Daisy were toddlers, Lisa and I have taken them on countless wilderness and city walks. To the playground, to the supermarket; footpaths beside lakes, bathing in the green blur. There is small talk, and there are big talks. Grievances are aired. Affection swells. Lisa collects sticks and leaves and rocks and flowers with the girls. As we cook dinner, our daughters make sculptures and collages on the kitchen floor with their loot. "Within the space of a few decades, the way children understand and experience nature has changed radically," Richard Louv writes in *Last Child in the Woods: Saving Our Children from Nature-Deficit Disorder*. "The polarity of the relationship has reversed. Today, kids are aware of the global threats facing their environment — but their physical contact, their intimacy with nature, is fading."

In May, I had brought Maggie and Daisy with me on a Jane's Walk, one of the thousands of free public walks offered around the world every year in honour of Jane Jacobs. It was a food-foraging excursion in a ravine a few blocks from our house. We munched on watercress and day lilies, probiotic burdock root (good to kick-start the eliminative organs after a winter of potatoes and carrots) and goutweed (good for gout). Our guide, herbalist Amber Westfall, pointed out trees that release the chemicals that are studied by scientists in Japan, and seeds that can be used to make a tea that helps with grief. "Plants connect you to your bioregion," she said. "To the world you inhabit. A real intimacy can develop. If people get a sense of this connection, then they start to feel stewardship and responsibility."

Daisy gave me a thumbs-up as she chewed on a garlic mustard leaf. "It was more interesting than I thought it would be," she said about the walk when it was finished.

It takes less than an hour to drive from Toronto to the Bruce Trail, but I have not been back since I was a kid. We pull off the highway and park on a side road. Our backpacks are stuffed with Nutella sandwiches, frozen water bottles and bathing suits; we have a reservation at a B&B eight miles away. A wooden staircase leads into the lush forest. The girls race up the steps like squirrels. This will be their longest walk yet.

Maggie and Daisy gorge on raspberries, hold out their palms to create landing pads for tiny black-and-white butterflies, and are enthralled by the view, a hazy panorama extending to the smokestacks of Hamilton Harbour (which, in the distance, resemble the ramparts of a storybook fortress). Daisy shimmies along a fallen tree that juts out over the edge of the escarpment. I warn her to stay back from the cliff. Maggie corrects me: "It's more of a ledge than a cliff, Dad."

In addition to discovering the flora and fauna of a valuable conservation corridor, my daughters get a physics lesson. What goes up must come down. We cross a road and descend into a deep, ancient valley. The girls scoot ahead in their running shoes; my heavy leather hiking boots slip on the muddy slope. Youth trumps experience, although Daisy has another theory: "Maybe it's because you're clumsy, Dad."

We rest on a wooden bridge at the bottom, listening to a burbling stream, and take advantage of this rare unhurried day together to talk about the meaning of life — and death.

Daisy informs me that she doesn't believe in reincarnation. When you die, your spirit goes to heaven, she says. It's a place in the clouds.

"This place is pretty right here," Maggie cuts in, stepping down from the bridge to the shore.

"What's hell?" Daisy asks.

"What do you think?" I say.

"Aren't heaven and hell," says Maggie, looking up from the stream, where she is fishing stones out of the shallows, "the same thing?"

Daisy spots a daddy longlegs on my hat, which captures her attention. Then she scampers to join her sister at the water's edge.

The next physics lesson doesn't go over so well. What comes down often must go up again. We begin a long, steep climb out of the ravine. The afternoon is hot and humid. The complaints begin. Not just from the girls. My shirt is soaked with sweat. There's no breeze. The mosquitoes find us. I bribe the girls onward with lollipops, licking the dirt off Daisy's after she drops it, and doing the same for Maggie when she "accidentally" loses her grip.

The sugar kicks in on an evergreen-lined trail along the rim of the escarpment. The girls sing camp songs, cartwheel, balance on logs. They dig potato bugs and ants out of rotting trees with sticks, and wash their dirt-streaked hands and faces in the cascade above a waterfall.

The sun slants. Moments linger.

When our legs are heavy from six hours on the trail, I point through the trees to the streets of a small town down below. Soon we are running around a splash pad in a shaded park — laughing, leaping, soaring. Ready for anything.

EPILOGUE

"The whole concatenation of wild and artificial things, the natural ecosystem as modified by people over the centuries, the built environment layered over layers, the eerie mix of sounds and smells and glimpses neither natural nor crafted — all of it is free for the taking, for the taking in. Take it, take it in, take in more every weekend, every day, and quickly it becomes the theater that intrigues, relaxes, fascinates, seduces, and above all expands any mind that's focused on it. Outside lies utterly ordinary space open to any casual explorer willing to find the extraordinary. Outside lies unprogrammed awareness that at times becomes directed serendipity. Outside lies magic."

— *John Stilgoe, historian, Harvard University*

"Remember, one of the main tenets of capitalism is to have the consumer filled with fear, insecurity, envy and unhappiness so that we can spend, spend, spend our way out of it and, dammit, just feel better for a little while. But we don't, do we? The path to happiness — and deep down, we all know this — is created by love, and being kind to oneself, sharing a sense of community with others, becoming a participant instead of a spectator, and being in motion. Moving. Moving around all day. Lifting things, even if it's yourself. Going for a walk every day will change your thinking and have a ripple effect."

— *Michael Moore, filmmaker*

Early October, late evening, the waxing moon a sliver from full. A 10-foot-long stack of cross-hatched split white cedar has been doused in gasoline and set on fire. Now it has burned down into a bed of red-hot embers. Tongues of flame dance on the coals, which radiate about 1,500° Fahrenheit, and plumes of grey smoke drift into the dark sky.

I am east of Ottawa at a rural retreat owned by the family that runs Canada's largest chain of kung fu schools. For the past two hours, as the wood snapped and crackled, 30 of us sat inside the adjacent pagoda listening to grandmaster Jacques Patenaude and his son Martin talk us through the ritual we are about to experience. "You have an incredible force inside you," said Jacques, a short, stocky Franco-Ontarian who transformed a youth of bare-knuckled barn fighting and motorcycle-gang mischief into a martial arts empire. "It is the exhilaration of living.

"Some people make prisons in their own minds, but if you know who you are and what you want — if you focus and avoid distractions — you can harness this power to do anything."

Wearing a black T-shirt with "from fear to power" written on front and "I walked on fire!" on the back, Jacques springs to and fro when he speaks, and has a penchant for quoting Bruce Lee. "The teacher tonight will be the fire," he told us. "We are only the providers."

People have walked on hot coals since at least 1200 BC. From Iron Age India and Taoist Japan to Eastern Orthodox festivals in present-day Greece, the practice has been considered a rite of passage, a test of faith or courage. A way to overcome your fears. Tolly Burkan brought it to North America in the 1970s, opening an institute for fire-walking education and research in California's Sierra Nevada mountains; self-help guru Tony Robbins was one of his early disciples. Robbins convinced Oprah to try it at one of his "Unleash The Power Within" seminars. She called her midnight walk "one of the most incredible experiences of my life."

Almost all of my fellow walkers train at one of the Patenaudes' 22 dojos in Ontario and Quebec. Most say they have come for "personal development," the same reason people gave me when I asked why they had joined Stanley Vollant's Innu Meshkenu journey. *"J'aime beaucoup le barbecue,"* quipped one participant. *"C'est mon cadeaux,"* said another, brought blindly by his brother without knowing the destination. "It's a symbolic way to help me tackle challenges in my relationships," a rangy young man offered. (Later, I would learn that he is one of the Patenaudes' star students, the winner of several mixed martial arts prison fights against inmates in Thailand.) A guy with a shaved head and piercing eyes drove all the way from Toronto to be here. "My life is a complete disaster," he said to me. "I have to do something. This can't hurt."

Actually, it can. *People have been seriously injured by participating in fire walking*, read the waiver that I signed upon entering the pagoda. *There is an inherent risk.*

I am here seeking metaphorical closure. Two years is a long time to focus on one project, but this book is nearly complete. I started in snow, passed through a mental fog, explored the urban jungle and braved the worlds of business and politics. I even ventured into an art gallery and a church. Now I am ready to cross a threshold. To confront my biggest opponent — myself.

"The coals are hot," Martin announces from outside through the open sliding door. *"Super hot."*

"How many people," Jacques asks with a wink, "are we going to burn tonight?"

We are capable of doing extraordinary things on our feet. For instance, tightrope walking. I stare longingly at people slack-lining in parks, but have not yet had a chance to try it. "The essential thing is simplicity," advises French funambulist Philippe Petit, who walked between the Twin Towers on a steel cable when the buildings were nearing completion in 1974, spending 45 minutes spellbindingly suspended 110 storeys above Manhattan. "That is why the long path to perfection is horizontal."

Nor have I experienced the sensation of serious barefoot walking. Our feet did not evolve to be clad in cushioned footwear with rubber soles. These deaden the muscles and make us strike with our heels, which can lead to injuries. When infants put on shoes, they walk faster and take longer steps; the long-term impacts on gait are unknown. Going barefoot is like travelling atop a pair of stethoscopes, a geologist I know told me after he completed a bootless mountain hike in the Yukon. A gravel path in the city reminds him of munching potato chips. Some people believe that "grounding," unhindered contact with the earth, draws electrons into the body, and that these tiny, negatively charged particles can help regulate our biological clocks and neutralize infection. (One of my brothers, a molecular biophysicist, calls this pseudoscientific nonsense.)

The benefits of walking backwards are more established. It is said to be good for the knees and the back, for balance and posture, and for cardiovascular health, and may help us stay mentally sharp by putting the brain in an unfamiliar trajectory.

The trajectories explored in this book, the stories contained herein, continue to unfurl. As of this writing, in the fall of 2014, most of the people I walked with are still making slow and steady progress.

Stanley Vollant came through Ottawa in October, the weekend of my fire walk, and I joined him for a stroll along the river to a rally on Parliament Hill. "My project is not a protest," he told me. "It's an affirmative walk, to help empower people." Vollant has expeditions planned through 2017, including a short summer trek from Akwesasne to Montreal. That will be the finish line for Innu Meshkenu, but later, who knows: maybe he'll head to Vancouver.

Rich Mitchell is collecting data for the Woodlands In and Around Town experiment in Scotland, and though the Glasgow effect remains a mystery, researchers in England have new evidence that the relationship between access to green space and reduced mortality is most pronounced in deprived areas.

Matt Green has covered more than 7,500 miles, but because he is spending so much time these days doing background research on the photos he posts to his website, and not actually walking, he doesn't expect to see every inch of every block in New York City until some point in 2018. On a recent afternoon, after a three-month drought, he spotted Headz Ain't Ready, his 92nd "barberz" shop, between a shoe store and a courier service for Colombian immigrants, on 37th Avenue in Queens.

Beat cops continue to patrol North Philadelphia, and one of the two men accused of killing police officer Moses Walker, Jr., has pled guilty to third-degree murder and agreed to testify against his co-defendant.

Neighbourhoods across Canada are starting to lose home delivery of mail, and a massive building on the Canada Post administrative campus near my house has a mural on its side: a Richard Long–sized painting of a smiling letter carrier with a shopping cart full of parcels. "Delivering the online world," reads the tagline. (The last time I passed by, that slogan was still there, but a new image depicted four shopping carts and no postie.)

Spence the basset hound is riding shotgun in Andrew Markle's car and has yet to have an accident in the vehicle.

Mike Collier's *Walk On* exhibition is still touring the U.K., and Todd Shalom has shifted Elastic City's focus to an annual festival of free walks.

In the home stretch of the Scottish independence referendum, MP Rory Stewart cancelled plans for a unifying hand-holding rally along Hadrian's Wall, the Roman fortification that shadows England's northern border in Cumbria. Instead, he walked the wall path for a couple of days, a landscape where people "had eaten olives, and gazed at the wet ground, and the scrub, and the distant line of hills, for 300 years."

My grandmother sold her condo and moved into an apartment in an assisted-living building. There is a tree-lined footpath around its perimeter, and she is now within walking distance of my parents' house.

Work has yet to begin on the textured brick crossing at the busy intersection near my daughters' school. But a large blue "information/guidance sign Mx-38" has been installed beside the pedestrian button at all four corners.

Even when I wasn't looking for walkers, I found them. In the crossroads village of Tamworth, Ontario, population 200, I rented a suite above a store for a week so I could have a quiet place to work. Three days before I arrived, a reclusive man, provoked by a dispute over muskrat trapping, had gone on a shooting spree, killing one person and sending two others to the hospital before taking his own life. During my stay, on a cold March night, almost everybody who lives in Tamworth gathered outside the hockey arena for a healing walk, a silent procession through the streets. "The violence happened over such a wide geographic area," one of the organizers said to me as we passed the post office, where a firefighter had been shot, "so there's a sense that we are taking back the space." The walk, she believed, would replace images of violence in the minds of locals with images of community.

A couple of months later, Lisa, the girls and I spent a weekend in a town called Bancroft, near Tamworth. In the park next to our hotel, an all-night Relay for Life cancer fundraiser was under way. As a band played classic rock songs on a stage decked out like a log cabin, men and women walked laps on a trail around the park boundary, their route lined by paper bags bearing names of — and messages for — cancer survivors and victims. I returned to the park after Maggie and Daisy were in bed. Lit up by electric candles, flickering in the dark grass, the "luminaries" looked magical, like small beacons that might at any moment float up into the sky. "Cancer fears the walker," somebody had written on one. There was a chill in the air. I did a lap to stay warm, and then another.

Glaciers are melting. The Middle East is exploding. Ebola is spreading. Why bother? Why walk? Why not withdraw behind walls, and travel on wheels or wings?

Because walking is a tonic for body, mind and soul. Because the act can restore health and inspire hope in places where there is not much of either. Because it can help replant the seeds of independence and interdependence, two things we cannot bloom without. Michael Pollan distilled his recipe for a healthy diet into seven simple words. *Eat food. Not too much. Mostly plants.* My manifesto fits into three. *Walk more. Anywhere.*

Wood is not a very good conductor of heat. When you walk across a bed of embers, your feet don't stay in contact with the coals long enough to burn. That's the theory, anyway. Jacques Patenaude has done it 300 times, distances up to 40 feet long, and has been singed six times.

"Don't look directly at the fire, and don't run," he told us. That pushes your feet deeper into the embers, and increases the likelihood of injury. "But don't go too slow," he added.

We line up on a rubber mat outside the pagoda. The sound of West African drumming and rhythmic clapping fills the air.

Martin rakes the coals, sending a shower of sparks into the night.

We are told to extend our arms forward, palms up, and to repeat the mantra "cool moss."

My mind is clear when I reach the edge of the fire. Nothing flashes in front of my eyes. No wave of emotion or fear. After an instant's hesitation, I simply step forward — "cool moss, cool moss" — and six footfalls later I am standing on the damp grass on the other side. There was a small pinch on the arch of my left foot, but no other pain. No strong sense of catharsis, either. Just the feeling that once I started, it was easier to keep moving than to stop.

When everybody in the group has walked through the coals, I circle around to the back of the line, ready to go again.

SOURCES

The majority of the interviews referenced below were completed specifically for this book. Others were simultaneously conducted for articles that were published in *The Walrus*, the *Globe and Mail*, *The Economist*, *enRoute*, *Canadian Business*, *Ottawa Magazine*, *Spacing*, *Cottage Life* and *explore*, where portions of the book have appeared.

PROLOGUE

"Perhaps walking is best imagined": Rebecca Solnit, *Wanderlust: A History of Walking* (Penguin, 2001), 250.

"I walk in order to somatically medicate myself": Will Self, "Leaving His Footprints on the City," *New York Times*, 23 March 2012.

"Mediated boredom": Evgeny Morozov, "Only Disconnect," *The New Yorker*, 28 October 2013.

"[A] state in which the mind, the body, and the world are aligned," Solnit, *Wanderlust*, 5.

"French philosopher Frédéric Gros": Frédéric Gros, *A Philosophy of Walking* (Verso, 2014).

"British author Nick Hunt": Nick Hunt, *Walking the Woods and the Water: In Patrick Leigh Fermor's Footsteps From the Hook of Holland to the Golden Horn* (Nicholas Brealey, 2014).

"Historian Matthew Algeo": Matthew Algeo, *Pedestrianism: When Watching People Walk Was America's Favorite Spectator Sport* (Chicago Review Press, 2014).

"Naturalist Trevor Herriot": Trevor Herriot, *The Road Is How: A Prairie Pilgrimage Through Nature, Desire and Soul* (HarperCollins Canada, 2014).

1: BODY

Interviews with Stanley Vollant and other Innu Meshkenu walk participants, February and March 2013, between Manawan, QC, and Rapid Lake, QC.

"Canada's 1.4 million Aboriginal people": www12.statcan.gc.ca/nhs-enm/2011/as-sa/99-011-x/99-011-x2011001-eng.cfm.

"Aboriginal men and women die an average": Statistics Canada, Life Expectancy, www.statcan.gc.ca/pub/89-645-x/2010001/life-expectancy-esperance-vie-eng.htm.

"Infant mortality rate": Assembly of First Nations, "Fact Sheet — Quality of Life of First Nations," June 2011, www.afn.ca/uploads/files/factsheets/quality_of_life_final_fe.pdf.

"Chronic medical condition": Health Canada, First Nations and Inuit Health, www.hc-sc.gc.ca/fniah-spnia/diseases-maladies/index-eng.php.

"First Nations children . . . overweight or obese": Public Health Agency of Canada, Obesity in Canada — Snapshot, www.phac-aspc.gc.ca/publicat/2009/oc/index-eng.php.

"A full-blown crisis": Heart and Stroke Foundation, "A perfect
storm of heart disease looming on our horizon," 25 January
2010, www.heartandstroke.com/atf/cf/{99452D8B-E7F1-
4BD6-A57D-B136CE6C95BF}/Jan23_EN_ReportCard.pdf.

"Statistics on . . . incarceration": Office of the Correctional
Investigator, Annual Report 2012–2013, www.oci-bec.gc.ca/cnt/
rpt/annrpt/annrpt20122013-eng.aspx.

"Most common cause of death": Health Canada, First Nations &
Inuit Health, www.hc-sc.gc.ca/fniah-spnia/promotion/mental/
index-eng.php.

"Youngest and fastest-growing demographic group": Statistics
Canada, Aboriginal Peoples in Canada, www12.statcan.gc.ca/
nhs-enm/2011/as-sa/99-011-x/99-011-x2011001-eng.cfm.

"Indian Time": Duncan McCue, Reporting in Indigenous
Communities, www.riic.ca/the-guide/in-the-field/
indian-time/.

Interviews with Jean-Charles Fortin, February and March 2013,
between Manawan, QC, and Rapid Lake, QC.

"Americans are in the habit": Jeff Speck, *Walkable City: How
Downtown Can Save America, One Step at a Time* (Farrar, Straus
and Giroux, 2012), 101.

"A pedometer study": Tom Vanderbilt, "The Crisis in American
Walking," *Slate*, 10 April 2012, www.slate.com/articles/life/
walking/2012/04/why_don_t_americans_walk_more_the_
crisis_of_pedestrianism_.html.

"The decline of walking": Vanderbilt, "The Crisis in American
Walking."

Tom Vanderbilt, *Traffic: Why We Drive the Way We Do (and What
It Says About Us)* (Vintage, 2008).

"London physiologist Richard Doll": Richard Doll and Austin
Bradford Hill, "Smoking and Carcinoma of the Lung:
Preliminary Report," *British Medical Journal* 2 (30 September
1950): 739–748.

"British health minister Iain Macleod": The National Archives,

The Cabinet Papers 1915–1984, www.nationalarchives.gov.uk/
cabinetpapers/themes/one-page.htm.

"London doctor Jerry Morris": Simon Kuper, "The Man Who
Invented Exercise," *FT Magazine*, 12 September 2009, www
.ft.com/intl/cms/s/0/e6ff90ea-9da2-11de-9f4a-00144feabdc0
.html#axzz3E3QFLQUS.

"Coronary Heart-Disease and Physical Activity of Work," Jerry
Morris, *The Lancet* 262, no. 6795 (November 1953): 1053–1057.

"Upright ambulation": Smithsonian National Museum of Natural
History, humanorigins.si.edu/human-characteristics/walking;
and Erin Wayman, "Becoming Human," *Smithsonian*, 6 August
2012, www.smithsonianmag.com/science-nature/becoming-
human-the-evolution-of-walking-upright-13837658/?no-ist.

"Using a stiff leg": Jennifer Ackerman, "The Downside of Upright,"
National Geographic, July 2006.

"The Brain from Top to Bottom": thebrain.mcgill.ca.

"Narrow birth canals": Ackerman, "The Downside of Upright."

"A lot of basic movements": Peter Tyson, "Our Improbably Ability
to Walk," NOVA, 20 September 2012, www.pbs.org/wgbh/
nova/body/our-ability-to-walk.html.

"Walking upright . . . made our species smarter": Richard Shine
and James Shine, "Delegation to automaticity: the driving force
for cognitive evolution?" *Frontiers in Neuroscience* 8, no. 90 (29
April 2014).

"Evolutionary compromises": Ackerman, "The Downside of
Upright."

"University College London . . . meta-analysis of walking research":
Harvard Health Publications, Harvard Medical School, "Walking:
Your steps to health," August 2009, www.health.harvard.edu/
newsletters/Harvard_Mens_Health_Watch/2009/August/
Walking-Your-steps-to-health.

"Emma Wilmot of the University of Leicester": Emma Wilmot
et al., "Sedentary time in adults and the association with diabetes, cardiovascular disease and death: systematic review

and meta-analysis," *Diabetologia* 55, no. 11 (14 August 2012): 2895–2905.

"These are sobering numbers": André Picard, "Why the sedentary life is killing us," *Globe and Mail*, 15 October 2012.

Interview with Michael Evans, telephone, April 2013.

Interview with Michael Vallis, telephone, April 2013.

"Globally, the number of overweight and obese people soared": "Global, regional, and national prevalence of overweight and obesity in children and adults during 1980–2013: A systematic analysis for the Global Burden of Disease Study 2013," *The Lancet* 384, no. 9945 (30 August 2014): 766–781.

"Forest bathing": Florence Williams, "Take Two Hours of Pine Forest and Call Me in the Morning," *Outside*, December 2012.

"*Shinrin-yoku*, a term introduced": Yoshifumi Miyazaki et al., "The physiological effects of *Shinrin-yoku* (taking in the forest atmosphere or forest bathing): evidence from field experiments in 24 forests across Japan," *Environmental Health and Preventive Medicine* 15, no. 1 (January 2010): 18–26.

"The presence of phytoncides": Yoshifumi Miyazaki, Qing Li et al., "Phytoncides (wood essential oils) induce human natural killer cell activity," *Immunopharmacology and Immunotoxicology* 28, no. 2 (February 2006): 313–333.

"Mice kept in a fragrant environment . . . reduced melanoma growth": M. Kusuhara et al., "Fragrant environment with α-pinene decreases tumor growth in mice," *Biomedical Research* 33, no. 1 (24 February 2012): 57–61.

"Middle-aged Japanese businessmen": Qing Li, "Effect of forest bathing trips on human immune function," *Environmental Health and Preventive Medicine* 15, no. 1 (January 2010): 9–17.

"It's like a miracle drug": Williams, "Take Two Hours."

"All human physiological functions": Yoshifumi Miyazaki et al., "Physiological effects of Shinrin-yoku (taking in the atmosphere of the forest) using salivary cortisol and cerebral activity

as indicators," *Journal of Physiological Anthropology* 26, no. 2
(February 2007): 123–128.

Interview with Margaret MacNeill, Toronto, April 2013.

Interviews at Toronto's Challenging Environment Assessment
Laboratory, November 2013.

"Sleep apnea": Harvard Medical School, "The Price of Fatigue:
The surprising economic costs of unmanaged sleep apnea,"
December 2010.

"The price we pay for falling": The iDAPT Centre, www.idapt.
com/index.php/labs-services/research-labs/ceal-labs/stairlab.

"One in three people over 65 falls every year in Canada": Vicky
Scott, Lori Wagar and Sarah Elliott, "Falls and Related Injuries
among Older Canadians," Public Health Agency of Canada, 30
April 2010, www.hiphealth.ca/media/research_cemfia_phac_
epi_and_inventor_20100610.pdf.

Interview with Amanda Boxtel, telephone, November 2013.

"Second most significant gadget of 2010": Gadget Lab Staff, *Wired*,
December 2012, www.wired.com/2010/12/top-tech-2010.

"Ask any wheelchair user": Red Nicholson, "Why the obsession
with walking?" Attitude Live, 5 June 2014, attitudelive.com/
blog/red-nicholson/opinion-why-obsession-walking.

2: MIND

"Right now, we are deciding": Elizabeth Kolbert, *The Sixth
Extinction: An Unnatural History* (Henry Holt and Co., 2014).

"I know of no thought so burdensome": Søren Kierkegaard, letter
to his niece Henriette Lund, 1847, quoted in *Kierkegaard: The
Indirect Communication*, Roger Poole (University of Virginia
Press, 1993), 172.

"Scotland has the lowest life expectancy": Office for National
Statistics, 16 April 2014, www.ons.gov.uk/ons/publications/
re-reference-tables.html?edition=tcm%3A77-354758.

"The Glasgow effect": Glasgow Centre for Population Health,

"Investigating a 'Glasgow Effect,'" April 2010, www.gcph.co.uk/
publications/61_investigating_a_glasgow_effect.

"Scottish Health Survey": Office for National Statistics, "The
Scottish Health Survey: The Glasgow Effect," November 2010,
www.scotland.gov.uk/Resource/Doc/330419/0107211.pdf.

"Just make a bloody start": Ali Muriel, "Mystery of
Glasgow's health problems," *The Guardian*, 6 November
2012, www.theguardian.com/society/2012/nov/06/
mystery-glasgow-health-problems.

"I had not walked farther than the golf house": Carl Lira,
"Biography of James Watt," www.egr.msu.edu/~lira/supp/
steam/wattbio.html.

"The start of the Anthropocene": Lee Billings, "Embracing the
Anthropocene," *Seed*, 19 March 2010, seedmagazine.com/
content/article/embracing_the_anthropocene.

Interviews with participants in the Paths for All/Scottish National
Heath Service health walk program, Glasgow, July 2013.

"Persistent loneliness": Mental Health Foundation, "The Lonely
Society?" 2010, www.mentalhealth.org.uk/content/assets/
PDF/publications/the_lonely_society_report.pdf.

"Social return on investment analysis": Paths for All, "Glasgow
Health Walks: Social Return on Investment Analysis," July 2013,
www.pathsforall.org.uk/sroi.

"With good company": Canadian Centre for Occupational Health
and Safety, "Walking: Still Our Best Medicine," 20 April 2006,
www.ccohs.ca/oshanswers/psychosocial/walking.html.

"Walking could help forestall brain shrinkage": Alan Gow et al.,
"Neuroprotective lifestyles and the aging brain," *Neurology* 79,
no. 17 (23 October 2012): 1802–1808.

"A healthy brain can slow the progression": Kirk Erickson,
"Physical activity predicts gray matter volume in late adult-
hood," *Neurology* 75, no. 16 (19 October 2010): 1415–1422.

"An estimated 5.2 million Americans had Alzheimer's": The

Alzheimer's Association, Facts and Figures, www.alz.org/
alzheimers_disease_facts_and_figures.asp#quickFacts.

Interview with Rich Mitchell, Glasgow, August 2013.

"Regular exercise in a park or forest may halve your risk": Richard
Mitchell, "Is physical activity in natural environments better for
mental health than physical activity in other environments?"
Social Science & Medicine 91 (August 2012): 130–134.

"The social determinants of health": World Health Organization,
"The Solid Facts," 2003, www.euro.who.int/__data/assets/
pdf_file/0005/98438/e81384.pdf.

"View Through a Window": Roger Ulrich, "View Through a
Window May Influence Recovery from Surgery," *Science* 224,
(1984): 420–421.

"Attention Restoration Theory": Rachel Kaplan and Stephen
Kaplan, *The Experience of Nature: A Psychological Perspective*
(Cambridge University Press, 1989).

"All fascinations are not equally effective": Rachel Kaplan, Stephen
Kaplan and Robert Ryan, *With People in Mind: Design and
Management of Everyday Nature* (Island Press, 1998), 18.

"Another American psychologist, Terry Hartig": Terry Hartig et
al., "Tracking restoration in natural and urban field settings,"
Journal of Environmental Psychology 23, no. 2 (June 2003): 109–123.

"The less vigorous activity of walking": Roma Robertson et al.,
"Walking for depression or depressive symptoms: a systematic
review and meta-analysis," *Mental Health and Physical Activity* 5,
no. 1 (June 2012): 66–75.

"Green space can reduce stress": Richard Mitchell et al., "More
green space is linked to less stress in deprived communities:
Evidence from salivary cortisol patterns," *Landscape and Urban
Planning* 105, no. 3 (April 2012): 221–229.

"Woods In and Around Towns": Richard Mitchell et al., "How
effective is the Forestry Commission Scotland's woodland
improvement programme . . . at improving psychological

well-being in deprived urban communities?" *BMJ Open*, August 2013.

Interview with Sean Gobin, telephone, October 2013, and information from warriorhike.com.

"The risk of exposure to trauma": Matthew Friedman, U.S. Department of Veterans Affairs, PTSD History and Overview, www.ptsd.va.gov/professional/PTSD-overview/ptsd-overview .asp.

"Distance changes utterly when you take the world on foot": Bill Bryson, *A Walk in the Woods: Rediscovering America on the Appalachian Trail* (Doubleday, 1996).

Interviews with Shauna Joye and Zachary Dietrich, telephone, December 2013.

"More than 350 million people globally suffer from depression": World Health Organization, October 2012, www.who.int/ mediacentre/factsheets/fs369/en.

"Preventing depression . . . a question of movement": Sarah Goodyear, "How Simple Physical Activity Could Stave Off Depression," CityLab, 13 February 2014, www.citylab.com/ commute/2014/02/how-simple-physical-activity-could-stave -depression/8398.

"Inactive mice are more anxious": Timothy Schoenfeld et al., "Physical exercise prevents stress-induced activation of granule neurons and enhances local inhibitory mechanisms in the dentate gyrus," *Journal of Neuroscience* 33, no. 18 (May 2013): 7770–7777.

"Walking is the cheapest and easiest way to get relief from depression": *The Walking Revolution*, everybodywalk.org/documentary

Interview with Mark Norwine, telephone, February 2014.

"Duke University neuroscientist James Blumenthal": James Blumenthal et al., "Exercise Treatment for Major Depression: Maintenance of Therapeutic Benefit at 10 Months," *Psychosomatic Medicine* 62, no. 5 (September/October 2000): 633–638.

Interview with Chuck Hillman, telephone, September 2013.

"A single 20-minute bout of exercise": Chuck Hillman et al., "The Effect of Acute Treadmill Walking on Cognitive Control and Academic Achievement in Preadolescent Children," *Neuroscience* 159, no. 3 (March 2009): 1044–1054.

"Children . . . diagnosed with ADHD": Centers for Disease Control and Prevention, ADHD Data & Statistics, www.cdc.gov/ncbddd/adhd/data.html.

"Pharmaceutical companies earned nearly $9 billion" and "psychologist Keith Connors": Alan Schwarz, "The Selling of Attention Deficit Disorder," *New York Times*, 14 December 2013.

"Something this simple could help wean us off Ritalin": Gordon Rayner, "Walking to school 'could help reduce need for ADHD drugs,'" *The Telegraph*, 26 September 2013.

"Chronic stress leads to inactivity": William Bird, "Combatting NCDs — Time to Get Moving," *The Economist*, 18 November 2013.

"A brief epidemic of hysterical fugue": Ian Hacking, *Mad Travelers: Reflections on the Reality of Transient Mental Illnesses* (University of Virginia Press, 1998).

"Nearly 30 percent of Europe's adult population": H.U. Wittchen et al., "The size and burden of mental disorders and other disorders of the brain in Europe 2010," *European Neuropsychopharmacology* 21, no. 9 (September 2011): 655–679.

3: SOCIETY

"The city is seen as serving a democratic function": Jan Gehl, *Cities for People* (Island Press, 2010), 109.

"If there is any way of seeing less of a country": Eric Newby, *A Short Walk in the Hindu Kush* (Secker and Warburg, 1958).

"Walker looked over his left shoulder": youtu.be/KJdK7PMVaB8.

Interviews with Philadelphia police officers and residents in the 22nd District, Philadelphia, June 2013.

"Being human is itself difficult": Jane Jacobs, *The Death and Life of Great American Cities* (Vintage, 1961), 447.

"The way you travel around a city impacts your impressions": Birgitta Gatersleben et al., "Hoody, goody or buddy? How travel mode affects social perceptions in urban neighbourhoods," *Transportation Research Part F: Traffic Psychology and Behaviour* 21 (November 2013): 219–230.

"Existential reassurance": Tim Kreider, "The 'Busy' Trap," *New York Times*, 30 June 2012.

"The city's murder capital": Philadelphia Police Department, "Murder/Shooting Analysis, 2013" www.phillypolice.com/assets/crime-maps-stats/HomicideReport-2013.pdf, 3.

"You stand on the corner, you fighting": Daniel Denvir, Samantha Melamed and Eric Schneider, "Dispatches from Killadelphia," *Philadelphia City Paper*, 26 September 2013.

"The 331 homicides committed in Philadelphia": Philadelphia Police Department, "Murder/Shooting Analysis, 2013."

"Manage the social conflict": George L. Kelling, "Juveniles and Police: The End of the Nightstick," *From Children to Citizens, Vol. II: The Role of the Juvenile Court*, ed. Francis X. Hartmann (Springer-Verlag, 1987).

"At first, all officers walked their beats in Philly": Howard O. Sprogle, *Philadelphia Police, Past and Present* (LBS Archival Products, 1992).

"I've always had a theory": Shaila Dewan, "As Gas Prices Rise, Police Turn to Foot Patrols," *New York Times*, 20 July 2008.

"Newark Foot Patrol Experiment": Police Foundation, 1981, www.policefoundation.org/content/newark-foot-patrol-experiment-report.

"Foot patrol . . . had been pretty much discredited": George L. Kelling and James Q. Wilson, "Broken Windows," *The Atlantic*, March 1982.

Interview with Jerry Ratcliffe, telephone, June 2013.

"Philadelphia Foot Patrol Experiment": Department of Criminal Justice, Temple University, www.temple.edu/cj/footpatrolproject.

"In a rough part of Rotterdam": "The Neighbourhood Takes

Charge," www.rotterdam.nl/factsheet_neigbourhood_takes
_charge_project and www.huffingtonpost.ca/jon-packer/
urban-crime_b_4959466.html.

Interview with Matt Green, Harlem, June 2013.

"To tear down all the generalizations": Matt Green, "Why I'm
Walking Every Single Block in New York City," *Good*, 24 March
2013, magazine.good.is/articles/why-i-m-walking-every-single-
block-in-new-york-city and imjustwalkin.com/nyc-details.

"Waves of immigration and gentrification": William B. Helmreich,
The New York Nobody Knows (Princeton University Press, 2013).

"When we think about cities," Matt Green at TEDxDumbo, 13
October 2012, youtu.be/XlR4fVGI39s.

"The enterprise and adventure of the day": Henry David Thoreau,
"Walking," *Atlantic Monthly*, June 1862.

"The pedestrian is nobody in this city": Nicholas Casey, "A Very
Pedestrian Superhero Grapples With Mexico City Traffic," *Wall
Street Journal*, 29 May 2013.

"About 270,000 pedestrians are killed by motor vehicles":
World Health Organization, "Global Status Report on road
Safety 2013," www.who.int/violence_injury_prevention/
road_safety_status/2013/en.

"More than 47,000 pedestrians were killed on American streets":
Smart Growth America, "Dangerous by Design 2014," www
.smartgrowthamerica.org/research/dangerous-by-design/
dbd2014/national-overview.

"Distracted driving . . . 1.6 million accidents": National Safety
Council, www.nsc.org/Pages/NSCestimates16million
crashescausedbydriversusingcellphonesandtexting.aspx.

"Everyone knows to look left and right": "Phones put pedestrians
in a fog," *Consumer Reports*, August 2012.

"Texting while walking not only distorts the flow of sensory
information": Siobhan Schabrun et al., "Texting and Walking:
Strategies for Postural Control and Implications for Safety,"
PLUS ONE 9 (January 2014).

"Disdain toward walking": Tom Vanderbilt, "The Crisis in American Walking."

"As far back as the 14th century BC": Leigh Gallagher, *The End of the Suburbs: Where the American Dream Is Moving* (Portfolio/Penguin, 2013).

"Dispersed cities were a capitalist's dream": Charles Montgomery, *Happy City: Transforming Our Lives Through Urban Design* (Doubleday, 2013).

"Rates of diabetes among baby boomers": interview with Dr. Michael Evans, telephone, April 2013.

"The farther people commute": Montgomery, *Happy City*.

"The social impact of commuting": Robert Putnam, *Bowling Alone: The Collapse and Revival of American Community* (Simon & Schuster, 2000), 213.

"A global, total obesity": Jeff Speck, *Walkable City: How Downtown Can Save America, One Step at a Time* (Farrar, Straus and Giroux, 2012), 101–102.

"Urban population growth . . . outpaced suburban growth": Leigh Gallagher, "The End of the Suburbs," *Time*, 31 July 2013.

"Sprawl subsidy": Naheed Nenshi, youtu.be/Eqszj5IYlV4.

"Death and injury on city streets": City of New York, "Vision Zero Action Plan 2014," www.nyc.gov/html/visionzero/pdf/nyc-vision-zero-action-plan.pdf.

"Copenhagen's 40-year-long evolution": Jan Gehl, *Cities for People* (Island Press, 2010).

"The book is a call to arms": Speck, *Walkable City*.

"People, this is Los Angeles": David Hochman, "Hollywood's New Stars: Pedestrians," *New York Times*, 16 August 2013.

"Annual quality-of-living survey": International HR Adviser, www.internationalhradviser.co.uk/storage/downloads/2012%20Quality%20Of%20Living%20Worldwide%20City%20Rankings%20Survey.pdf.

"A comforting signal that people are nearby": Gehl, *Cities for People*, 99.

"Limit parking and require density": Donald Shoup, *The High Cost of Free Parking* (Planners Press, 2005).

"In one of the first research projects of its kind": Jane Farrow and Paul Hess, "Walkability in Toronto's High-Rise Neighbourhoods," Cities Centre, University of Toronto, 2010.

"Walking environments are not simply routes from A to B": "Walkability in Toronto's High-Rise Neighbourhoods," 5.

"Women's walking is often construed as performance": Solnit, *Wanderlust*, 234.

"A video that went viral": youtu.be/b1XGPvbWn0A.

"Nearly half of all women are afraid of walking alone at night": General Social Survey, 1972–2012, National Opinion Research Center, www3.norc.org/gss+website.

"A poem by John Morse": www.nyc.gov/html/dot/downloads/pdf/curbside-haiku-sample.pdf.

"Not one of those kids": Associated Press, "Chicago Homicides Down Drastically in 2013 to Fewest Murders Since 1965, Police Say," 1 February 2014, www.huffingtonpost.com/2014/01/02/chicago-homicides-down-dr_n_4531328.html.

4: ECONOMY

"In exchange for profit and speed": Melanie Mackenzie, "Canada Post wants to eliminate my job as a letter carrier. Here's why you should care," *The Coast*, 19 December 2013.

"All the fancy economic development strategies": Christopher Leinberger, *The Option of Urbanism: Investing in a New American Dream* (Island Press, 2009), 170.

Interview with Christine Murray, Ottawa, November 2013.

"Benign symbol of the larger web of governance": "Post Office Symbolism," *New York Times*, 23 July 2003.

"Pen-named postie": Bill Walker, "The Last Post?" *The Walrus*, May 2012.

"Facing a 25 percent decrease in mail volume": The Conference

Board of Canada, "The Future of Postal Service in Canada," April 2013.

"The corporation made a profit": "Canada Post: Mail volume, costs, and other quick facts," CBC News, 11 December 2013, www.cbc.ca/m/touch/news/story/1.2459693.

"The United States Postal Service": USPS, "A decade of facts and figures," about.usps.com/who-we-are/postal-facts/decade-of-facts-and-figures.htm.

"Royal Mail posted a pre-tax profit": Ian Walker, "Royal Mail Posts Strong Profit Growth in First Annual Results Since IPO," *Wall Street Journal*, 22 May 2014.

"The world's largest online retailer": "Amazon Booms in 2013 with $74.45 Billion in Revenue," 30 January 2014, www.digitalbook world.com/2014/amazon-booms-in-2013-with-74-45-billion-in-revenue.

"You're sort of like a robot": Sarah O'Connor, "Amazon Unpacked," *FT Magazine*, 8 February 2013, www.ft.com/intl/cms/s/0/ed6a985c-70bd-11e2-85d0-00144feab49a.html#slide0.

"A call for insider stories": Hamilton Nolan, "True Stories of Life as an Amazon Worker," *Gawker*, 2 August 2013, gawker.com/true-stories-of-life-as-an-amazon-worker-1002568208.

"The blue-collar British town of Rugeley": O'Connor, "Amazon Unpacked."

"Walking levels fell 66 percent": Alliance for Biking & Walking, "Bicycling and Walking in the United States, 2012 Benchmarking Report," 2012, www.bikewalkalliance.org/resources/benchmarking#previousreports.

"The cost of obese and overweight citizens": Society of Actuaries/Committee on Life Insurance Research, "Obesity and Its Relation to Mortality and Morbidity Costs," December 2010.

"Let's go retro, folks": U.S. Surgeon General Boris Lushniak, *Washington Post* Health Beyond Health Care Forum, 18 June 2014, www.washingtonpost.com/blogs/post-live/wp/2014/06/24/surgeon-general-walking-and-cooking-are-your-patriotic-duties.

"As economic recession has hit almost every level of our society":
Alliance for Biking & Walking, "Bicycling and Walking," 174.

"Transportation infrastructure work in Baltimore": Heidi Garrett-
Peltier, Political Economy Research Institute University of
Massachusetts, "Estimating the employment impacts of pedes-
trian, bicycle, and road infrastructure, case study: Baltimore," 2010.

Chris Turner, *The Leap: How to Survive and Thrive in the Sustainable
Economy* (Random House, 2011).

"58 construction projects in 11 American cities": Garrett-
Peltier, Political Economy Research Institute University of
Massachusetts, "Pedestrian and Bicycle Infrastructure: A
National Study of Employment Impacts," June 2011.

"Complete Streets": www.smartgrowthamerica.org/
complete-streets.

"A walkable community also raises property values": Downtown
Baltimore Family Alliance, "Enhancing Walkability in the City
of Baltimore," May 2011, dbfam.org/PDF/DBFA_Walkability_
White_Paper.pdf, 4.

"A one-point Walk Score increase will boost housing values": Joe
Cortright, "Walking the Walk: How Walkability Raises Home
Values in U.S. Cities," CEOs for Cities, August 2009.

"Consumer spending in British towns": Todd Litman, Victoria
Transport Policy Institute, "Economic Value of Walkability,"
22 March 2014, 15, www.vtpi.org/walkability.pdf.

"Six in 10 Americans say they would choose": National
Association of Realtors, "2011 Community Preference
Survey," 18 March 2011, 2, www.realtor.org/
reports/2011-community-preference-survey.

"Walkability is more than an attractive amenity": Richard Florida,
"America's Most Walkable Cities," *The Atlantic*, 15 December 2010.

"The city an hour down the highway": Christopher Leinberger
and Mariela Alfonzo, Brookings Institution, "Walk This Way:
The Economic Promise of Walkable Places in Metropolitan
Washington, D.C.," 25 May 2012.

"The car has . . . at the centre of our transportation policies":
Litman, "Economic Value of Walkability."

"The personal cost savings from reduced vehicle use": Litman,
"Economic Value of Walkability."

"Portland, Oregon . . . an urbanist poster child": Joe Cortright,
"Portland's Green Dividend," CEOs for Cities, July 2007.

Interview with Jennifer Keesmaat, Toronto, November 2013.

"In Wales, walking . . . puts food on the table": Economy Research
Unit, Cardiff University, "The Economic Impact of Walking
and Hill Walking in Wales," 28 June 2011.

"About 2.9 million people walked on the wcp": Economy Research
Unit, Cardiff University, "The Economic Impact of Wales Coast
Path Visitor Spending on Wales 2012," November 2012.

"Difficult to associate monetary values to biodiversity and landscape":
"The Economic Impact of Walking and Hill Walking in Wales," 3.

Interview with Joseph Murphy, New Galloway, Scotland, July 2013.

"Poorly conceived development projects": Joseph Murphy, *At
the Edge: Walking the Atlantic Coast of Ireland and Scotland*
(Sandstone Press, 2009).

"All economic activity is dependent upon that environment":
Gaylord Nelson, *Beyond Earth Day: Fulfilling the Promise*
(University of Wisconsin Press, 2002).

"Greenhouse-gas emissions in the U.S.": United States
Environmental Protection Agency, National Greenhouse Gas
Emissions Data, www.epa.gov/climatechange/ghgemissions/
usinventoryreport.html.

"The first mile of my walk is just a racket": Dan Pallotta, "Take a
Walk, Sure, but Don't Call it a Break," *Harvard Business Review*
Blog Network, 27 February 2014, blogs.hbr.org/2014/02/
take-a-walk-sure-but-dont-call-it-a-break.

"Management by walking around": "Management by walking
about," *The Economist*, 8 September 2008.

"You can take care of your health": Nilofer Merchant, "Got a

meeting? Take a walk," TED Talk, February 2013, on.ted.com/
   Nilofer.

Interview with Margaret MacNeill, Toronto, April 2013.

"An intricate argument under time pressure": Daniel Kahneman,
   Thinking, Fast and Slow (Doubleday, 2011).

"Chairdom is hugely effecting humans": Susan Orlean, "The
   Walking Alive," *New Yorker*, 20 May 2013.

"The effectiveness of working while on a treadmill": Dinesh
   John, David R. Bassett et al., "The Effect of Using a Treadmill
   Workstation on Performance of Simulated Office Work,"
   Journal of Physical Activity & Health 6, no. 5 (September 2009):
   617–624.

Interview with Brecken Hancock and Andrew Markle, Ottawa,
   February 2014.

5: POLITICS

"Is a democracy, such as we know it": Henry David Thoreau, "Civil
   Disobedience," 1849.

"I learnt how distant my colleagues and I in government": Rory
   Stewart, "My long march to be a Tory MP in Cumbria," *The
   Sunday Times*, 3 January 2010.

Interview with Rory Stewart, Penrith and Tebay, U.K., July 2013.

"The expressions of the farmers": Rory Stewart, "My long march."

"Dead ringer for one or more of the Rolling Stones": *Vanity Fair*,
   "Hunky Foreign Correspondents and How to Woo Them,"
   8 February 2013, www.vanityfair.com/politics/2013/02/
   hottest-male-foreign-correspondents_slideshow_item1_2.

"One of the 75 most influential people of the 21st century": Parag
   Khanna, "Rory Stewart," *Esquire*, 6 October 2008, www.esquire
   .com/features/75-most-influential/rory-stewart-1008.

"It's just a phenomenally bad end to a film": Decca Aitkenhead,
   "Rory Stewart: 'The secret of modern Britain is there is no
   power anywhere,'" *The Guardian*, 3 January 2014.

"A dreamlike disconnection with the world": Julian Glover, "Rory Stewart's awfully big adventure," *The Guardian*, 14 January 2010.

"Backward, peripheral, and irrelevant": Rory Stewart, *The Places in Between* (Harvest/Harcourt, 2006), 25.

"There are three metres of snow": Stewart, *The Places in Between*, 3.

"The only piece of foreign technology was a Kalashnikov": Stewart, *The Places in Between*, xii.

"Al-Qaeda was good at the beginning": Stewart, *The Places in Between*, 84.

"Because the Russian government": Stewart, *The Places in Between*, 143.

"I was passed like a parcel down the line": Stewart, *The Places in Between*, 207.

"The creation of a centralized, broad-based multiethnic government": Stewart, *The Places in Between*, 245.

"A serious study of an alien culture": Stewart, *The Places in Between*, 247.

"Stewart is far too independent": Ian Dunt, "Rory Stewart's remarkable Commons speech showed how to make the case for the union," 6 February 2014, www.politics.co.uk/comment-analysis/2014/02/06/rory-stewart-s-remarkable-commons-speech-showed-how-to-make.

"Even a familiar walk . . . can provide new perspectives": Henry David Thoreau, "Walking," *The Atlantic*, June 1862, www.theatlantic.com/magazine/archive/1862/06/walking/304674.

"The Women's Suffrage Parade": Alan Taylor, *The Atlantic*, 3 March 2013, www.theatlantic.com/infocus/2013/03/100-years-ago-the-1913-womens-suffrage-parade/100465.

"White legs and negro legs": Taylor Branch, *The King Years: Historic Moments in the Civil Rights Movement* (Simon & Schuster, 2013), 66.

"Next to sex": Eric Hobsbawm, *Interesting Times: A Twentieth-Century Life* (Allen Lane, 2002) 73.

"Another leap forward": Branch, *The King Years*.

"American Indian Movement": www.aimovement.org/ggc/history.html.

"Prof. Lehman Brightman": youtu.be/086w-erjlgQ.

"The complex intersections of desert ecology, human health and
     culture": Susie O'Brien, "Survival Strategies for Global Times:
     The Desert Walk for Biodiversity, Health and Heritage,"
     Interventions: International Journal of Postcolonial Studies 9, no. 1
     (2007): 84–99.

Interview with Leanne Simpson, telephone, April 2013.

"The Native Women's Walk to Ottawa": Janet Silman, *Enough Is
     Enough: Native Women Speak Out* (Women's Press, 1992).

"We really didn't think anybody would listen to us": *Enough Is
     Enough*, 162.

"First Nations' grandmothers": Kevin McMahon, "A native grand-
     mother's epic walk for the water," *Toronto Star*, 4 April 2009.

Interview with Leo Baskatawang, April 2013.

"Hereditary chief Beau Dick": Jeffrey Jones, "Idle No More: March
     to Victoria," *Sointula Ripple*, 13 February 2013, sointularipple
     .ca/2013/02/idle-no-more-march-to-victoria.

Interview with Ben Isitt, telephone, April 2014.

Interview with Dave Sauchyn, telephone, October 2013.

Interview with John Fraser, Ottawa, July 2013.

"One of the most remarkable lives on record": Anna van Praagh,
     "Rory Stewart: A new kind of Tory," *The Telegraph*, 1 November
     2009.

"Politics as we have known it totters": The Dark Mountain
     Manifesto, dark-mountain.net/about/manifesto.

6: CREATIVITY

"Walking exposes us to the constant flux": Paul Sowden, National
     Trust, www.ntsouthwest.co.uk/tag/weekend-walk.

"I can only meditate when I am walking": Jean-Jacques Rousseau,
     Confessions, 1782.

Interview with Todd Shalom and Ben Weber, Brooklyn, June 2013.

"Suspensive freedom": Frédéric Gros, *A Philosophy of Walking*
     (Verso Books, 2014), 5.

"Aristotle walked back and forth": William Clark, *Academic Charisma and the Origins of the Research University* (University of Chicago Press, 2007), 71.

"Diogenes . . . *solvitur ambulando*": Arianna Huffington, "Hemmingway, Thoreau, Jefferson and the Virtues of a Good Long Walk," 29 August 2013, www.huffingtonpost.com/arianna-huffington/hemingway-thoreau-jeffers_b_3837002.html.

"One of his hikes through a concealed pass": Michael Michalko, "Thought Walking," 19 November 2012, www.creativitypost.com/create/thought_walking.

"William Wordsworth . . . some 180,000 miles": Solnit, *Wanderlust*, 104.

"By being forced to focus on quick-passing logistical realities": Trina-Marie Baird, "How did walking serve as an integrative activity for Wordsworth?" (Lancaster University, Dept. of Religious Studies, 2008).

"Nietzsche maintained an equally disciplined schedule": Drake Baer, "The workday secrets of the world's most productive philosophers," *Fast Company*, 9 October 2013, www.fastcompany.com/3019654/leadership-now/the-workday-secrets-of-the-worlds-most-productive-philosophers.

"Only thoughts reached by walking have value": Friedrich Nietzsche, *Twilight of the Idols*, 1889.

"Richard Long took a train southeast": www.tate.org.uk/art/artworks/long-a-line-made-by-walking-ar00142/text-summary.

"Long changed our notion of sculpture": Sean O'Hagan," One Step Beyond," *The Observer*, 10 May 2009, www.theguardian.com/artanddesign/2009/may/10/art-richard-long.

"Anywhere": www.richardlong.org/Textworks/2012textworks/anywhere.html.

"Internal horizon line, craggy and rugged": British Council, visualarts.britishcouncil.org/exhibitions/exhibition/out-of-britain-2012/object/spring-circle-long-1992-p6284.

"A walking definition of humanity": Laura Cumming, "Hamish
Fulton: Walk, Turner and the Elements — review," *The
Guardian*, 29 January 2012, www.theguardian.com/artanddesign
/2012/jan/29/hamish-fulton-walk-turner-margate-review.

"Slowalk (In support of Ai Weiwei)": www.turnercontemporary
.org/news/hamish-fulton-slowalk-in-support-of-ai-weiwei.

"Only art resulting from the experience of individual walks":
www.tate.org.uk/whats-on/tate-britain/exhibition/
hamish-fulton-walking-journey.

"A passive protest against urban societies": British Council,
visualarts.britishcouncil.org/collection/artists/hamish-fulton-
1946/initial/f.

Interview with Mike Collier, Sunderland, U.K., July 2013.

*"Walk On: From Richard Long to Janet Cardiff — 40 Years of Art
Walking"*: Cynthia Morrison-Bell, Mike Collier, Tim Ingold,
Alistair Robinson, official catalogue (Art Editions North, 2013).

"Jena Walk (Memory Field)": www.cardiffmiller.com/artworks/
walks/jena.html.

"I get it from, like, walking around": youtu.be/10wl-Fipvtk.

"The country's not that wide": www.artgarfunkel.com/articles/
talks.html.

"Walk Rule No. 1: No peeking": Tom Dunkel, "He's gone to look
for America," *Sports Illustrated*, 15 October 1990.

"The impact of walking in nature on creative problem-solving":
Ruth Ann Atchley and David Strayer, "Creativity in the Wild:
Improving Creative Reasoning through Immersion in Natural
Settings," *PLoS ONE*, 12 December 2012.

"Awesomely Adaptive and Advanced Learning and Behavior
unit": Marily Oppezzo and Daniel L. Schwartz, "Give Your
Ideas Some Legs: The Positive Effect of Walking on Creative
Thinking," *Journal of Experimental Psychology* 40, no. 4 (April
2014): 1142–1152.

Interview with Marily Oppezzo, telephone, April 2014.

"The dual process theory of cognition": Kahneman, *Thinking, Fast and Slow*.

"A torrent of new information": Sowden, www.ntsouthwest.co.uk/tag/weekend-walk.

Interview with Paul Sowden, telephone, March 2014.

Interview with Liane Gabora, telephone, April 2014.

"The 'big bang' of creativity": Liane Gabora, *The Cambridge Handbook of Creativity* (Cambridge University Press, 2010), 279–301.

"Painter Ryan Larkin": National Film Board, 1968, www.nfb.ca/film/walking/.

"I stepped from one word to the next": Stephen King, "On Impact," *The New Yorker*, 19 June 2000.

"The Pedestrian": Ray Bradbury, "The Pedestrian," *The Golden Apples of the Sun* (Doubleday, 1953).

7: SPIRIT

"Pilgrimages make it possible": Solnit, *Wanderlust*, 50.

"If you walk hard enough": Bruce Chatwin, *In Patagonia* (Penguin Classics, 2003), 43.

Interviews on the Llŷn Peninsula, Wales, August 2013.

"The rain and wind are hard masters": R.S. Thomas, "Too Late," *Collected Poems: 1945–1990* (Phoenix Press, 2002).

"A liminal state, between past and future identities": Solnit, *Wanderlust*, 51.

"Transforming ordinary life into a continuous practice of meditation": John Cianciosi, "Mindful Nature Walking (One Step at a Time)," *Yoga Journal*, 28 August 2007, www.yogajournal.com/article/practice-section/mindful-nature-walking-one-step-at-a-time.

"About 95 percent of the time": Francis Tapon, "10 Reasons Why El Camino Santiago Sucks," francistapon.com/Travels/Spain-Trails/10-Reasons-Why-El-Camino-Santiago-Sucks.

"Pilgrims typically depart feeling serene and blissful": Stephen
Reicher, "Participation in Mass Gatherings Can Benefit Well-
Being: Longitudinal and Control Data from a North Indian
Hindu Pilgrimage Event," *PLoS ONE*, 17 October 2012.

"The power of collective experience": Stephen Reicher, "Kumbh
Mela festival is proof that crowds can be good for you," *The
Guardian*, 15 January 2013, www.theguardian.com/science/
blog/2013/jan/15/kumbh-mela-festival-crowds-good-for-you.

"In this space you can achieve a direct human interaction": eds.
Ellen Badone and Sharon R. Roseman, *Intersecting Journeys:
The Anthropology of Pilgrimage and Tourism* (University of Illinois
Press, 2004).

"Ritual experiences that represent breaks": Gideon Lewis-Kraus,
A Sense of Direction: Pilgrimage for the Restless and the Hopeful
(Riverhead Books, 2012).

"Humanity, with fearful, faltering steps": www.peacepilgrim.com/
htmfiles/mdppbio.htm.

"They have a sustainable way of life": Andrew Chung, "Montreal
man walks around the world," *Toronto Star*, 1 October 2011,
www.thestar.com/news/canada/2011/10/01/montreal_man_
walks_around_the_world.html.

"Inching slowly across the surface of the earth": Naomi Sharp, "On
the job," *Columbia Journalism Review*, 2 January 2014, www.cjr
.org/on_the_job/on_the_job_1.php.

"Why aren't more people giving away everything": "Self-
Improvement Kick," *This American Life*, 1 April 2013, www.this
americanlife.org/radio-archives/episode/483/transcript.

"My years as the know-it-all naturalist": Herriot, *The Road Is How*.

"Milquetoast Harold Fry": Rachel Joyce, *The Unlikely Pilgrimage of
Harold Fry* (Random House, 2012).

"In many ways, the Pennine Way is a pointless exercise": Simon
Armitage, *Walking Home: Travels with a Troubadour on the Pennine
Way*" (Faber and Faber, 2012).

8: FAMILY

"Let children walk with nature": John Muir, *A Thousand-Mile Walk to the Gulf* (Houghton Mifflin, 1916), xii.

"We're so marinated in the culture of speed": Carl Honoré, *In Praise of Slow* (Vintage, 2004).

"The best time to talk to your kids": "Fire, Water, Earth, Air: Micahel Pollan Gets Elemental in 'Cooked,'" 21 April 2013, www.npr.org/2013/04/21/177501735/fire-water-air-earth-michael-pollan-gets-elemental-in-cooked.

"Unconscious synchronicity — an indicator of social interaction": Shinsuke Shimojo, Kyongsik Yun and Katsumi Watanabe, "Interpersonal body and neural synchronization as a marker of implicit social interaction," *Scientific Reports*, 11 December 2012.

"Shared feelings of rapport": Daniël Lakens and Mariëlle Stel, "If They Move in Sync, They Must Feel in Sync: Movement Synchronicity Leads to Attributions of Rapport and Entitativity," *Social Cognition* 29 (2011): 1–14.

Interview with Carl Honoré, telephone, June 2014.

"In the U.S., 89 percent of students": U.S. Department of Transportation, "Nationwide Personal Transportation Survey" (1972), www.fhwa.dot.gov/ohim/1969/q.pdf.

"Today, 35 percent cover that short distance": The National Center for Safe Routes to School, "How Children Get to School: School Travel Patterns from 1969 to 2009," saferoutesinfo.org/sites/default/files/resources/NHTS_school_travel_report_2011_0.pdf.

"Number of kids shuttled to school in personal vehicles": Safe Routes to School, "Children's Mobility, Health and Happiness: A Canadian School Travel Planning Model," www.saferoutestoschool.ca/downloads/Executive%20Summary-CLASP%20Results-May%202012.pdf.

"In its 2014 report card": Active Healthy Kids Canada, "Is Canada in the Running?," dvqdas9jty7g6.cloudfront.net/reportcard2014/AHKC_2014_ReportCard_Short_ENG.pdf.

"Harried parenting and rampant materialism": Adriana Barton,
"Consumerism is creating cunning and callous kids, therapist
finds," *Globe and Mail*, 29 May 2014, www.theglobeandmail
.com/life/parenting/consumerism-is-creating-cunning-and-
callous-kids/article18913979.

"The power to transform relationships": Roman Krznaric, *Empathy:
A Handbook for Revolution* (Random House, 2014).

"Kids who travel predominantly on foot": Sarah Goodyear, "Kids
Who Get Driven Everywhere Don't Know Where They're
Going," CityLab, 7 May 2012, www.citylab.com/commute/
2012/05/kids-who-get-driven-everywhere-dont-know-where
-theyre-going/1943.

"Frequently expressed feelings of dislike and danger": Bruce
Appleyard, "Livable streets for schoolchildren," www.india-
seminar.com/2013/648/648_bruce_appleyard.htm.

"People who live on city streets with lighter traffic have more
friends": Donald Appleyard, *Livable Streets* (University of
California Press, 1981).

"Cars are happiest": Dan Burden, Project for Public Spaces,
www.pps.org/reference/dburden.

"The walk to school is also a right of passage": Jennifer
Keesmaat, TEDxRegina, 16 May 2012, www.tedxregina.com/
video-gallery-2012.

Interview with Jennifer Keesmaat, Toronto, November 2013.

"Busyness has acquired social status": Brigid Schulte, *Overwhelmed:
Work, Love, and Play When No One Has the Time* (Sarah Crichton
Books, 2014).

"Canada's first master-planned suburb": Noor Javed, "Toronto's
mother of all suburbs," *Toronto Star*, 21 March 2009, www.the
star.com/news/gta/2009/03/21/torontos_mother_of_all_
suburbs_don_mills.html.

"The area around Peanut Plaza": Jane Farrow and Paul Hess,
"Walkability in Toronto's High-Rise Neighbourhoods," Cities
Centre, University of Toronto, 2010.

"Although these roads were conceived": Farrow and Hess, "Walkability in Toronto's High-Rise Neighbourhoods," 2.

"A continual fulfilled life": Emily Smith, "Walking as a way of life," American Trails, www.americantrails.org/resources/health/wayoflife.html.

"You feel like a twosome": Howard Scott, "Walk with her," *Boston Globe*, 19 February 2012, www.bostonglobe.com/magazine/2012/02/19/walk-with-her/zuZerB9IrEqyOBpm1QGrVL/story.html.

"High-visibility crossings": Ann McGrane and Meghan Mitmann "An Overview and Recommendations of High-Visibility Crosswalk Marking Styles," Pedestrian and Bicycling Information Center, for U.S. Federal Highway Administration, katana.hsrc.unc.edu/cms/downloads/PBIC_WhitePaper_Crosswalks.pdf.

"LPI signals": National Association of City Transportation Officials, *Urban Street Design Guide* (Island Press, 2013), 128.

Interviews at Queen Elizabeth Public School, Ottawa, May 2014.

"Lower-income households": Ontario Ministry of Education, www.edu.gov.on.ca/eng/sift/schoolProfile.asp?SCH_NUMBER=463523.

"Pedestrian collisions are tied with car accidents": Linda Rothman et al., "Walking and child pedestrian injury: a systematic review of built environment correlates of safe walking," *Injury Prevention* 20, no. 1 (February 2014): 41–49.

"A rise in child pedestrian collisions": Linda Rothman, "Motor Vehicle-Pedestrian Collisions and Walking to School: The Role of the Built Environment," *Pediatrics*, published online 7 April 2014.

"Ontario's education ministry spends": Green Communities Canada, "Saving Money and Time With Active School Travel," September 2010, www.saferoutestoschool.ca/oldsite/downloads/Saving_Money_and_Time_with_AT-Final-Sept_2010.pdf.

"The number of schools participating in STP-like programs": National Center for Safe Routes to School, "Trends in Walking and Bicycling to School from 2007 to 2012," October 2013,

saferoutesinfo.org/sites/default/files/Trends_in_Walking_
and_Bicycling_to_School_from_2007_to_2012_FINAL.pdf.
"Founder Ray Lowes envisioned": "Ray Lowes, Father
of the Bruce Trail, 1911–2007," brucetrail.org/news/
show/9-ray-lowes-father-of-the-bruce-trail-1911-2007.
"Within the space of a few decades": Richard Louv, *Last Child
in the Woods: Saving Our Children from Nature-Deficit Disorder*
(Algonquin Books, 2008), 1.
Interview with Amber Westfall, Ottawa, May 2013.

EPILOGUE
"The whole concatenation of wild and artificial things": John
Stilgoe, "The Art of the Everyday Adventure," *Utne Reader*
(from the book *Outside Lies Magic*), July–August 1999, www
.utne.com/mind-and-body/plainadventures.aspx.
"Remember, one of the main tenets of capitalism": Michael
Moore, "Why I walk," www.michaelmoore.com/
walk-with-mike.
Interviews with Jacque Patenaude and others at the Fang Shen Do
fire walk, Casselman, Ontario, October 2014.
"One of the most incredible experiences of my life": Marianne
Schnall, "Tony Robbins Sets the Record Straight About Fire
Walk 'Controversy,'" *Huffington Post*, 31 July 2012, www
.huffingtonpost.com/marianne-schnall/tony-robbins-fire-
walk_b_1718499.html.
"The essential thing is simplicity": "Etching Movements in the Sky,"
The Alchemist's Pillow, 11 September 2011, www.alchemists
pillow.com/2011/09/etching-movements-in-sky.html.
"Long-term impacts on gait": Caleb Wegener et al., "Effect of chil-
dren's shoes on gait: a systematic review and meta-analysis,"
Journal of Foot and Ankle Research, 18 January 2011, www.jfoot
ankleres.com/content/4/1/3.
"Grounding,' unhindered contact with the earth": James L.
Oschman, "Can electrons act as antioxidants? A review and

commentary," *The Journal of Alternative and Complementary Medicine* 13, no. 9 (November 2007): 955–967.

"The benefits of walking backwards": Joseph Mercola, "Stimulate your fitness IQ by walking backwards," 14 December 2012, fitness.mercola.com/sites/fitness/archive/2012/12/14/walking-backward.aspx.

Interview with Stanley Vollant, Ottawa, October 2014.

"Researchers in England have new evidence": Kate Lachowycz and Andy P. Jones, "Does walking explain associations between access to greenspace and lower mortality?" *Social Science & Medicine* 107 (15 February 2014): 9–17.

"Headz Ain't Ready": Matt Green, imjustwalkin.com/2014/04/20/barberz-92.

"Had eaten olives, and gazed at the wet ground": Rory Stewart, "Rory Stewart walks Hadrian's Wall," *Financial Times*, 20 June 2014, www.ft.com/intl/cms/s/2/7bd1ed92-f318-11e3-a3f8-00144feabdc0.html#axzz3H1dN5wEB.

"A reclusive man, provoked by a dispute over muskrat trapping": Joe Friessen and Claude Scilley, "Shootings leave tiny Southern Ontario town of Tamworth shaken," *Globe and Mail*, 28 February 2014.

Interviews in Tamworth, Ontario, March 2014.

"Wood is not a very good conductor of heat": John Roach, "Why fire walking doesn't burn: Science or spirituality?" *National Geographic News*, 1 September 2005, news.nationalgeographic.com/news/2005/09/0901_050901_firewalking.html.

ACKNOWLEDGEMENTS

Dozens of people have let me walk beside them and/or patiently answered my interminable questions over the past few years. This book would not have been possible without their generosity and wisdom. Most of their names appear in these pages already, and many should be mentioned again.

In Quebec, Stanley Vollant, Jean-Charles Fortin and Jesse Schnobb, who set the tone for my entire journey; in Glasgow, Rich Mitchell, Heather MacLeod and the members of the New Victoria Hospital health walk group; in Philadelphia, Sgt. Bisarat Worede and the foot patrol officers of the 22nd District; in New York City, Matt Green, who is doing so much more than "just" walking; in southwestern Scotland, geographer Joseph Murphy; in Ottawa, letter carrier Christine Murray, dog walkers Brecken Hancock and Andrew Markle, school travel activist Wallace Beaton, kung fu grandmaster Jacques Patenaude and Member of Provincial Parliament John Fraser; in England's Lake District, Member of Parliament Rory Stewart and legendary guide Chris Wright, who led me on an unforgettable hike to the top of Helvellyn; in Brooklyn, journalist Norman Oder and Todd Shalom and Ben Weber of Elastic City; in Sunderland, U.K., Mike Collier, who changed the way I think about art; in Wales, outfitter Peter Hewlett, who made sure all I had to worry about was walking; and in Tamworth, Ontario, Carolyn Butts and Hans Honegger, whose heritage apartment, creative energy and loaner snowshoes made for a fantastic writing retreat.

My extraordinary agent, Martha Magor Webb of Anne McDermid & Associates, was an enthusiastic supporter from the start. So was Kevin Patterson, whose passion for embarking on and writing about long walks sent me down this trail.

The team at ECW Press has been wonderful to work with and essential every step of the way: editor Jen Knoch was complimentary and critical in the right way, at the right time; co-publishers Jack David and David Caron gave me the freedom to say what I wanted; sales and marketing director Erin Creasey got the book out into the world; publicist Sarah Dunn and social media specialist Alexis Van Straten convinced people to read it; art director Rachel Ironstone gave it the right look and feel; designer David Gee nailed the cover; copy editor Stuart Ross caught my mistakes; and managing editor Crissy Calhoun kept us on track throughout the entire process.

Several magazines sent me on trips and/or published stories that were vital building blocks. Thank you to Amy Macfarlane at *The Walrus*, Deb Cummings and Jill Foran at *Up!*, Julie Traves at the *Globe and Mail*, Robert Guest at *The Economist*, Ilana Weitzman at *enRoute*, Natasha Mekhail at Spafax, David Fielding at *Canadian Business*, Rebecca Caldwell and Jay Teitel at *Cottage Life*, James Little at *explore*, Matthew Blackett and Dylan Reid at *Spacing*, and Sarah Brown and Dayanti Karunaratne at *Ottawa Magazine*. Other writer

and editor friends have provided invaluable advice and encourage-
ment: Rick Boychuk, Eric Harris, Alan Morantz, Allan Casey, Curtis
Gillespie, Chris Turner, Marcello Di Cintio, Scott Messenger, Craille
Maguire Gillies and many more whose names I have surely neglected to mention. (My bad!)

I lean heavily on several books in this work, in particular the
Rebecca Solnit classic *Wanderlust*, Jeff Speck's indispensable *Walkable
City*, Charles Montgomery's thought-provoking *The Happy City* and
Trevor Herriot's deeply moving *The Road Is How*. I urge you to read
them all.

The Canada Council for the Arts, Ontario Arts Council and
Canadian Institutes of Health Research provided much appreciated
grant funding.

To all my friends and family — especially my parents, my grandmother, my brothers and their families — thank you for steering
me in the right direction, and for listening to me rant about walking
with good humour.

And last, but most certainly not least, thank you to my daughters,
Maggie and Daisy, and to my wife, Lisa Gregoire, the best writer I
know, for allowing this project to share our home and our lives.

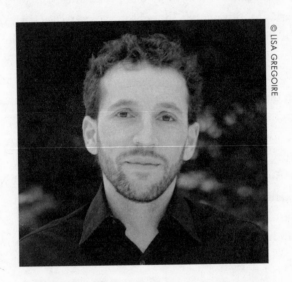

DAN RUBINSTEIN is a National Magazine Award–winning writer and editor. He contributes to publications such as *The Walrus*, the *Globe and Mail*, *The Economist* and *enRoute*, and has edited magazines in Ontario and Alberta. These days, he does most of his walking in Ottawa.